Busy People's Diabetic Cookbook

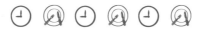

Dawn Hall

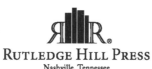

RUTLEDGE HILL PRESS
Nashville, Tennessee
A Division of Thomas Nelson Publishers
Since 1798

www.thomasnelson.com

To my friend, Nancy Roach,
for whom I have the utmost respect and admiration, I
dedicate this book. Her gentle spirit, sweet smile, and
kindness towards others, despite her daily challenges
with diabetes, are an inspiration to me.

I also dedicate this to my special Down's syndrome friend,
Esmie, who has diabetes. I love you, sweetheart! Just
thinking of you makes me happy!

Published by Rutledge Hill Press, a Division of Thomas Nelson, Inc., P.O. Box 141000, Nashville, Tennessee, 37214.

Rutledge Hill Press books may be purchased in bulk for educational, business, fundraising, or sales promotional use. For information, please email SpecialMarkets@ThomasNelson.com.

Library of Congress Cataloging-in-Publication Data

Hall, Dawn.
    Busy people's diabetic cookbook/Dawn Hall.
        p. cm.
    Includes index.
    ISBN 1-4016-0188-X (wirebound hardcover) 1. Diabetes—Diet therapy—Recipes.
2. Quick and easy cookery. I. Title.
    RC662.H338 2005
    641.5'6314--dc22

                                                        2004022811

Printed in China

05 06 07 08 09—5 4 3 2

Complete Your Busy People's Library

The recipes in these cookbooks are all easy to prepare and cook. They all contain 7 ingredients or less and can be prepared in less than 30 minutes.

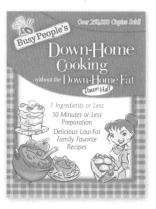

1-4016-0104-9
$16.99

1-4016-0215-0
$16.99
(Available May 2005)

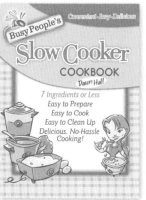

1-4016-0107-3
$16.99

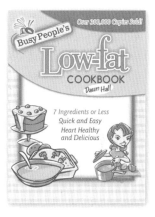

1-4016-0105-7
$16.99

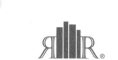

RUTLEDGE HILL PRESS
Nashville, Tennessee
A Division of Thomas Nelson Publishers
Since 1798

www.thomasnelson.com

**Available at better book stores everywhere!
or at www.RutledgeHillPress.com**

Contents

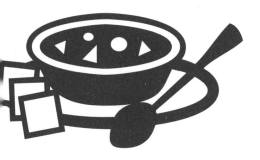

For more information about Dawn Hall

and her incredible journey, please consider this great
title from Harvest House Publishers

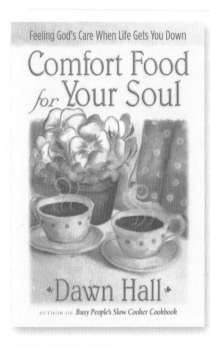

ISBN: 0-7369-1334-3
$9.99

When Dawn Hall's husband was diagnosed with cancer, her personal journey required total reliance on God and His comfort. Now she shares the discoveries she made during times of struggle and loss. Each brief chapter provides a slice of Dawn's insight, God's biblical recipes for hope, questions for reflection, and some of Dawn's favorite comfort food recipes.

Those seeking solace and kindness will be served gentle wisdom.

- **Stir It Up:** Experience how God moves in your life
- **Let Things Set:** Wait upon the Lord's faithfulness
- **Lick the Spoon:** Taste restoration and healing

For anyone experiencing loss or trials,
this book offers a taste of God's main ingredients for
all of us: hope, love, joy, and great faith.

(www.harvesthousepublishers.com)

Available at fine bookstores everywhere
or at www.amazon.com

Acknowledgments

My first debt of gratitude is to God. He has richly blessed me with the gifts and talents it takes to put a cookbook together. I'd be a fool to take credit for the creative ideas He gives me. I know it is He who gets all the praise and glory for each and every one of the great and wonderful things that happen through me.

Next, I am deeply grateful to those who helped me successfully create this book. I could not have done it alone. I am forever grateful to each of the following whose significant contributions led to the quality and high standards this cookbook delivers.

Dr. Thomas Knecht, you're not only an excellent doctor who specializes in diabetes, but you also live with diabetes. That is why you were my choice to write the foreword for this cookbook. I am honored to have your support and contribution to this cookbook. Thank you!

To my family, friends and personal assistants who continue being my taste testers, trying new ideas day in and day out without ever complaining, I give special thanks. Your brutal honesty motivates me to strive for the finest tasting recipes I can produce. Thank you for giving me the pat on the back for new recipes well done and a kick in the pants when you think I should go back to the kitchen and try again.

To Tammi Hancock, the registered dietician with over fifteen years experience who analyzed each and every recipe with perfection, much thanks for your feedback, insight and professional opinion on the recipes. I deeply appreciate all of your hard work each step of the way. Many thanks!

My Literary Agent, Coleen O' Shea, to whom I am forever grateful, thank you for being a better literary assistant than I could ever have hoped for, dreamed of, or imagined. You are a gem in my treasure chest of life. I will be forever grateful to JoAnna Lund, of Healthy Exchanges Cookbooks for introducing us to each other.

Brenda Crosser, my recipe-tester assistant, gets full credit for her creative ideas that were very good and inspired me to create more.

To Geoff Stone, my editor, who has a sharp eye for detail, thank you for polishing my work so it shines bright, crisp, and clean.

To Larry Stone, the publisher of Rutledge Hill Press, thank you for keeping the lines of communication open with me. Not all authors are as fortunate as I am to have such a great publisher. I want you to know I appreciate you.

To Bryan Curtis and Laura Troup, thank you for your marketing and publicity work in spreading the word.

Last but not least, I personally want to let you, *the reader,* know how incredibly grateful I am for letting your friends, family, and coworkers know how much you love using my cookbooks and how delicious the recipes taste. Word of mouth has been selling my *Busy People's* cookbooks like hotcakes because of you. Thank you from the bottom of my heart!

May God bless you always in all ways!

Foreword

I was diagnosed with type 1 diabetes in the 1970s when I was in college. My mom, who was a nurse, and my dad, who had no medical background (but was a brilliant guy), visited me for a weekend, saw that I was very sick, and said, "Tom, see a doctor!" I did and was directly admitted to the hospital.

This was before blood glucose testing, and I was first trained to use tablets to test glucose in urine. In retrospect, what a waste of time and resources! I was given instruction in diet, which at the time emphasized more a relationship to blood sugar than to overall health—the dark ages in diabetes management!

Things have come a long way since then. I actually have had the opportunity to live many of the advances that let us manage diabetes as successfully as we can today. I now use multiple meters, stationed in key locations (kitchen, office, briefcase, wife's purse, clinic, and others) that give me the blood glucose result in five to fifteen seconds (depending on the meter) using a tiny drop of blood. As an aggressive type 1 who wants excellent control with minimal serious hypoglycemia, I average about ten tests per day every day, and even more under certain circumstances.

You have this book in your hands, so likely you have diabetes or know someone very well who does. Type 1 diabetes (which usually occurs before adulthood) is an autoimmune disorder, which nothing can prevent—you stop producing the insulin that lets you use the food you eat and must inject insulin daily. In type 2 diabetes, you still make insulin to some degree, but for various reasons it isn't adequate. The cause of this type of diabetes is multifactorial and still somewhat elusive, but can be influenced by how you eat and exercise and by other factors. Type 2 once occurred primarily in adults, but is now increasingly being seen in children. You may be able to control type 2 diabetes with diet alone or with oral medications, and, in some cases, insulin is required.

The word *diabetes* actually has its root in "honeyed urine" first described in an ancient Hindu document from about 400 B.C. In 1922, the discovery of insulin was the single largest revolution in the timeline of diabetes in human medicine. (For one of the finest pieces of writing ever on the subject, turn to Michael Bliss' outstanding book, *The Discovery of Insulin*.) The march forward in diabetes therapy and management continued with the availability in the 1950s of the first oral medications for type 2 diabetes. Scientific and medical progress has continued, with the dawn of home blood glucose monitoring in the late 1970s (with tremendous refinement since then), to most recently newer categories of oral therapies for type 2 diabetes and to bioengineered insulins.

But before the industrial revolution of the eighteenth, nineteenth, and twentieth centuries, type 2 diabetes was essentially unknown. Since then type 2 diabetes has grown to the point that many more people have it than type 1 diabetes: from 1997 to 2000 alone, the rate of diabetes jumped 25 percent. Why? Partly because we are eating more refined sugar, refined flour, and highly saturated fat—at home and while eating out. (Check out the book *Fast Food Nation: the Dark Side of the All-American Meal*, by Eric Schlosser.) We've also become largely sedentary, another contributing factor. (Some of the recipes in this book call for refined, all-purpose flour because of the ease of availability. Although it is okay in moderation, the better way is to use whole wheat flour, which can be purchased at most large grocery stores or at specialty stores. You can substitute whole wheat flour for any recipe in this book.)

Both types of diabetes share the risk of serious complications: eye disease and blindness, kidney failure, and nerve damage that can cause severe pain and can contribute to the risk of amputation of the feet. These are the "microvascular" chronic complications of diabetes, and you can help lessen the risk by controlling your diabetes (through careful meal planning, among other things) and by controlling high blood pressure. People with type 2 diabetes also are at particularly high risk for "macrovascular" complications such as heart disease and heart attack, stroke, and hardening of the arteries to the kidneys and to the legs (which increases the risk of amputations). These problems are influenced by many factors: high cholesterol, diabetes, high blood pressure, smoking, metabolic factors, genetics, and others. These risks are very real, and every day that you do not take charge of your diabetes and these other risk factors increases the chances of these serious complications.

The good news is that better diabetes control in both types of diabetes can dramatically lessen if not eliminate the risk of complications. I am living proof that diabetes can be successfully managed. (And cutting calories, losing weight, eating less fat and more fiber, and getting regular exercise can play a vital role in avoiding type 2 diabetes altogether). I have seen treatment of type 2 diabetes come from using one category of oral agent and/or the older insulins, to now having four categories of oral agents that may be used in combination and/or the new insulin analogs, as well as aggressive management of their blood pressure and cholesterol. Throughout all this nothing-short-of-amazing progress, as a society, we have become more obese, less active, and more stretched for time. Bottom line, progress has not been across the board, and as a society we have regressed in some vitally important ways. We've come full circle to once again needing to strongly incorporate diet and exercise into our lifestyles.

So diet does matter—for both types of diabetes—and the book you hold in your hands can make eating well completely painless. Dawn Hall has put together a collection of more than two hundred tasty and easy-to-prepare healthy recipes, none with more than seven ingredients, that take only thirty minutes or less to prepare—and will appeal to the entire family. Your life is busy, and it may always seem easier to sit on the couch with take-out food or microwave snacks. But with only a little effort and planning, you can have a kitchen well-stocked with healthy foods, and can prepare tasty, healthful meals every day.

Your doctor can supply you with tools to help manage your diabetes. But only you can make the life commitment to living healthy, and can help yourself, friends, and family to value your health above most other things. Medicines alone are not enough: It is up to you to take control of your diabetes—and your life! This book is an excellent step in the right direction.

Thomas P. Knecht, MD, PhD, FACP
Division of Endocrinology
University of Utah School of Medicine
2004

To help you take control of your diabetes, it is my privilege and honor to share a special family recipe, one of my all-time favorites, from my mom. Admittedly it takes longer than a half hour to bake (about 35 minutes) and has more than seven ingredients—so it doesn't quite meet the criteria for this cookbook—but in this case I think the extra time and added ingredients are worth the additional effort. I know you are going to love it every bit as much as I do!

Peg Knecht's Healthy Gingerbread

3 cups whole wheat flour
3/4 cup sugar
I cup Splenda Granular
4 teaspoons ground ginger
4 teaspoons baking soda
5 egg whites

3/4 cup molasses
1/2 cup (I stick) reduced-fat margarine, melted*
I cup boiling water
1/2 cup no-sugar-added natural applesauce

- Preheat the oven to 350 degrees.
- Spray a 9 x 13-inch glass casserole dish with nonfat cooking spray.
- In large mixing bowl stir together the flour, sugar, Splenda, ginger, and baking soda until well mixed.
- Beat the egg whites in a large mixing bowl with an electric mixer on high speed until stiff peaks form.
- Add the molasses, melted margarine, applesauce, and boiling water to the beaten egg whites. Continue beating on medium-high speed with the mixer until well blended.
- Slowly add the dry ingredients and mix with the mixer on medium speed until well combined.
- Pour the batter into the prepared glass casserole dish.
- Bake for 35 minutes or until a toothpick inserted into the center comes out clean. This tastes best fresh and hot from the oven.

Note: To help with cholesterol use Smart Balance Light with no trans fat.

Yield: 16 servings

Calories: 188 (10% fat); Total Fat: 2 gm; Cholesterol: 0 mg; Carbohydrate: 40 gm; Dietary Fiber: 3 gm; Protein: 4 gm; Sodium: 369 mg
Diabetic Exchanges: 1 starch, 1 1/2 other carbohydrate

Introduction

My goal when creating this *Busy People's Diabetic Cookbook* was to have recipes with seven or less easy-to-find grocery store ingredients that diabetics and their families would both thoroughly enjoy eating. All Americans will benefit from this style of eating, not just diabetics.

If you are like me and were born watching your weight, I encourage you to start eating the diabetic way. You will be glad you did! Your health will improve and you will lose weight.

About the Ingredients

Some of you may be wondering why I didn't use only whole grain pastas, mixes, et cetera. In an ideal world we would all eat only whole foods that were grown in a garden full of nutrient-rich soil without any chemicals. The only vegetables and fruits we'd eat would be ones we had just picked from our gardens. Everything would be made from scratch with the freshest of ingredients, and we'd never eat anything that was processed.

However, that is not reality for most of us. For the most part, when it comes to eating, people want things easy. I even go so far as to say the easier the better. When preparing meals we need to take into consideration not only the time of cutting, chopping, peeling, preparing, and cooking the meal, but also the cleanup time afterwards, the shopping beforehand, and last but not least, the expense of the foods we eat.

If your local grocer has a good health food section you can afford, I encourage you, by all means, to buy the whole wheat pastas and cake mixes, fresh fruits and vegetables, et cetera and substitute them in my recipes for the easier-to-find grocery store ingredients. I tell my children this: we can have it all sometimes, but we can't have it all all the time. It just isn't realistic. That's why I have created these diabetic recipes and the menu ideas as I have. The recipes are designed with today's busy people in mind who want to be able to do all their shopping in one store, as quickly, affordably, and painlessly as possible, with their cooking to follow suit.

About Portion Sizes

When dieting and eating healthy, it is important to remember portion sizes. Eating low-fat foods is a great step in the right direction. However, simply eating these recipes without watching the size of your portions will not be enough. You need to watch portion sizes as well! It is also important to watch your side dishes. It is self-defeating if you eat a small portion of chicken Parmesan and then pig out on a loaf of garlic bread too. The entire consumption of all the foods and beverages you consume make up the balance of your diabetic diet for the day.

I've created menu ideas with the recipes that will help guide you in your meal creations. All the recipes are from my Busy People's cookbooks, and they all are easy and healthy. So, please, I encourage you. If you don't know about how to eat the diabetic way, read the information enclosed in this book. It is very helpful, informative, and user-friendly.

About Brand Names

Ground Meatless

Morningstar Farms Ground Meatless crumbles are low-fat, cholesterol-free burger crumbles. They are a taste equivalent to ground beef without all the fat. You can use these "crumbles" like cooked ground beef in all of my recipes. Ground Meatless crumbles are a textured vegetable protein product that contains wheat and soy ingredients. (They are found in the frozen food section of your local grocery store.)

Splenda

Splenda is a calorie-free sugar substitute that tastes like sugar and is made from sugar but without the fattening carbohydrates. I use it in a lot of my recipes.

There are two forms of Splenda: Splenda Granular and Splenda packets. Splenda Granular comes in a box and measures like sugar. Be careful when following my recipes that you use the appropriate type of Splenda. The two different forms measure differently and are not interchangeable.

Support Groups

I have found it quite helpful to have an accountability partner or support group in maintaining a healthy lifestyle with eating. There are many to choose from. Some groups, such as Weight Watchers, you have to pay to join. And there are free support groups, such as Body for Life. Programs with prepackaged foods can also be good.

Overeaters Anonymous is helpful in the accountability department, but I found some groups to be too focused on one area and lacking in other areas. The diabetic support groups at hospitals are wonderful. They cover dietary needs and requirements along with exercise.

Of all the groups, though, I have found the free group First Place to be the most comprehensive for me. It covers the overall well-being of the entire person, including the physical, spiritual, emotional, mental, and psychological. There is accountability, encouragement and support on all levels. You will receive as much or as little support as you desire. You will learn to eat appropriate portion sizes and to eat from all food groups; real food for real people. A healthy amount of exercise is encouraged as well as quiet time with God.

I cannot recommend First Place highly enough! For more information on First Place go to *www.Firstplace.org* or call 800-727-5223. You will be glad you did!

If you are diabetic, I strongly encourage you to talk with a medical professional who specializes in diabetes to oversee and set up an appropriate eating and lifestyle plan for you.

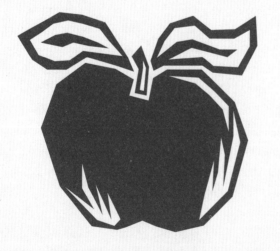

What You Need to Know about Eating & Diabetes

How food affects your blood glucose

Whether you have type 1 or type 2 diabetes, what, when, and how much you eat all affect your blood glucose. Blood glucose is the main sugar found in the blood and the body's main source of energy.

- If you have diabetes (or impaired glucose tolerance), your blood glucose can go too high if you eat too much. If your blood glucose goes too high, you can get sick.

- Your blood glucose can also go too high or drop too low if you don't take the right amount of diabetes medicine.

- If your blood glucose stays high too much of the time, you can get heart, eye, foot, kidney, and other problems. You can also have problems if your blood glucose gets too low (hypoglycemia).

- Keeping your blood glucose at a healthy level will prevent or slow down diabetes problems. Ask your doctor or diabetes teacher what a healthy blood glucose level is for you.

Blood glucose levels

What should my blood glucose levels be?

For most people, target blood glucose levels are

Before meals	**90 to 130**
1 to 2 hours after the start of a meal	**less than 180**

Ask your doctor how often you should check your blood glucose. The results from your blood glucose checks will tell you if your diabetes care plan is working. Also ask your doctor for an A1C test at least twice a year. Your A1C number gives your average blood glucose for the past three months.

How can I keep my blood glucose at a healthy level?

- Eat about the same amount of food each day.

- Eat your meals and snacks at about the same times each day.

- Do not skip meals or snacks.

- Take your medicines at the same times each day.

- Exercise at about the same times each day.

Why should I eat about the same amount at the same times each day?
Your blood glucose goes up after you eat. If you eat a big lunch one day and a small lunch the next day, your blood glucose levels will change too much.

Keep your blood glucose at a healthy level by eating about the same amount of carbohydrate foods at about the same times each day. Carbohydrate foods, also called carbs, provide glucose for energy. Starches, fruits, milk, starchy vegetables such as corn, and sweets are all carbohydrate foods. Talk with your doctor or diabetes teacher about how many meals and snacks to eat each day.

Your diabetes medicines
What you eat and when affects how your diabetes medicines work. Talk with your doctor or diabetes teacher about the best times to take your diabetes medicines based on your meal plan.

Your exercise plan

What you eat and when also depend on how much you exercise. Exercise is an important part of staying healthy and controlling your blood glucose. Physical activity should be safe and enjoyable, so talk with your doctor about what types of exercise are right for you. Whatever kind of exercise you do, here are some special things that people with diabetes need to remember:

- Take care of your feet. Make sure your shoes fit properly and your socks stay clean and dry. Check your feet for redness or sores after exercising. Call your doctor if you have sores that do not heal.

- Drink about 2 cups of water before you exercise, about every 20 minutes during exercise, and after you finish, even if you don't feel thirsty.

- Warm up and cool down for 5 to 10 minutes before and after exercising. For example, walk slowly at first, then walk faster. Finish up by walking slowly again.

- Test your blood glucose before and after exercising. Do not exercise if your fasting blood glucose level is above 300. Eat a small snack if your blood glucose is below 100.

- Know the signs of low blood glucose (hypoglycemia) and how to treat it.

Hypoglycemia

You should know the signs of hypoglycemia (low blood sugar) such as feeling weak or dizzy, sweating more, noticing sudden changes in your heartbeat, or feeling hungry. If you experience these symptoms, stop exercising and test your blood glucose. If it is 70 or less, eat one of the following right away:

- 2 or 3 glucose tablets
- $1/2$ cup (4 ounces) of any fruit juice
- $1/2$ cup of a regular (not diet) soft drink
- 1 cup (8 ounces) of milk
- 5 or 6 pieces of hard candy
- 1 or 2 teaspoons of sugar or honey

After 15 minutes, test your blood glucose again to find out whether it has returned to a healthier level. Once blood glucose is stable, if it will be at least an hour before your next meal, it's a good idea to eat a snack.

To be safe when you exercise, carry something to treat hypoglycemia, such as glucose tablets or hard candy. Another good idea is to wear a medical identification bracelet or necklace (in case of emergency). Teach your exercise partners the signs of hypoglycemia and what to do about it.

The food pyramid

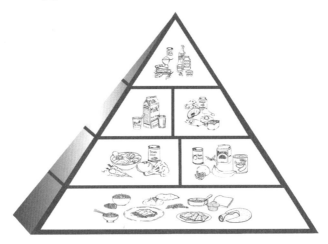

Eat a variety of foods to get the vitamins and minerals you need. Eat more from the groups at the bottom of the pyramid, and less from the groups at the top.

How much should I eat each day?

Have about 1,200 to 1,600 calories a day if you are

- a small woman who exercises
- a small or medium woman who wants to lose weight
- a medium woman who does not exercise much

Have about 1,600 to 2,000 calories a day if you are

- a large woman who wants to lose weight
- a small man at a healthy weight
- a medium man who does not exercise much
- a medium to large man who wants to lose weight

Have about 2,000 to 2,400 calories a day if you are

- a medium to large man who does a lot of exercise or has a physically active job
- a large man at a healthy weight
- a large woman who exercises a lot or has a physically active job

Starches

Starches are bread, grains, cereal, pasta, or starchy vegetables like corn and potatoes. They give your body energy, vitamins, minerals, and fiber. Whole grain starches are healthier because they have more vitamins, minerals, and fiber.

Eat some starches at each meal. People might tell you not to eat starches, but that is not correct. Eating starches is healthy for everyone, including people with diabetes.

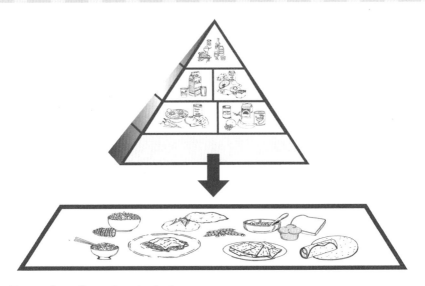

Examples of starches include

- bread
- pasta
- potatoes
- rice
- tortillas
- beans
- corn
- crackers
- yams

How much is a serving of starch?
Examples of 1 serving:

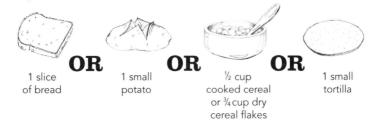

1 slice
of bread

OR

1 small
potato

OR

½ cup
cooked cereal
or ¾ cup dry
cereal flakes

OR

1 small
tortilla

Examples of 2 servings:

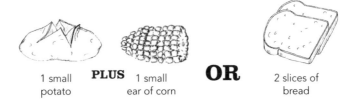

1 small
potato

PLUS

1 small
ear of corn

OR

2 slices of
bread

Examples of 3 servings:

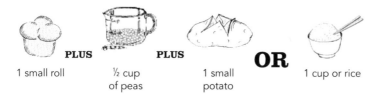

PLUS		**PLUS**	**OR**	
1 small roll	½ cup of peas	1 small potato		1 cup or rice

If you have more than one serving at a meal, you can choose several different starches or have two or three servings of one starch.

What are healthy ways to eat starches?

- Buy whole grain breads and cereals.

- Eat fewer fried and high-fat starches such as regular tortilla chips and potato chips, French fries, pastries, or biscuits. Try pretzels, fat-free popcorn, baked tortilla or potato chips, baked potatoes, or low-fat muffins.

- Use low-fat or fat-free yogurt or fat-free sour cream instead of regular sour cream on a baked potato.

- Use mustard instead of mayonnaise on a sandwich.

- Use the low-fat or fat-free substitutes such as low-fat mayonnaise or light margarine on bread, rolls, or toast.

- Eat cereal with fat-free (skim) or low-fat (1%) milk.

Vegetables

Vegetables give you vitamins, minerals, and fiber, with very few calories.

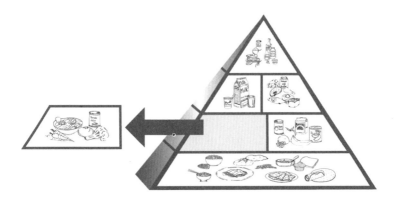

Examples of vegetables include

- lettuce
- broccoli
- vegetable juice

- peppers
- carrots
- green beans

- salsa
- chilies
- greens

How much is a serving of vegetables?
Examples of 1 serving:

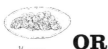 **OR** **OR**

½ cup cooked carrots

½ cup cooked green beans

1 cup salad

Examples of 2 servings:

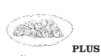 **PLUS** **OR** **PLUS**

½ cup cooked carrots

1 cup salad

½ cup vegetable juice

½ cup cooked green beans

Examples of 3 servings:

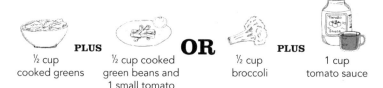

| ½ cup cooked greens | **PLUS** | ½ cup cooked green beans and 1 small tomato | **OR** | ½ cup broccoli | **PLUS** | 1 cup tomato sauce |

If you have more than one serving at a meal, you can choose a few different types of vegetables or have two or three servings of one vegetable.

What are healthy ways to eat vegetables?

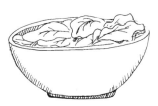

- Eat raw and cooked vegetables with little or no fat, sauces, or dressings.

- Try low-fat or fat-free salad dressing on raw vegetables or salads.

- Steam vegetables using a small amount of water or low-fat broth.

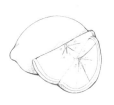

- Mix in some chopped onion or garlic.

- Use a little vinegar or some lemon or lime juice.

- Add a small piece of lean ham or smoked turkey instead of fat to vegetables when cooking.

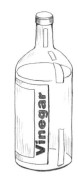

- Sprinkle with herbs and spices. These flavorings add almost no fat or calories.

- If you do use a small amount of fat, use canola oil, olive oil, or soft margarines (liquid or tub types) instead of fat from meat, butter, or shortening.

Fruit

Fruit gives you energy, vitamins, minerals, and fiber.

Examples of fruit include

- apples
- raisins
- bananas
- strawberries
- mangos
- oranges
- papayas
- guavas

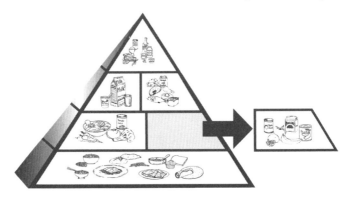

How much is a serving of fruit?
Examples of 1 serving:

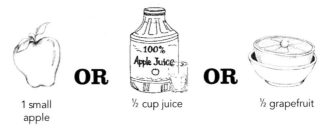

OR

OR

1 small
apple

½ cup juice

½ grapefruit

Examples of 2 servings:

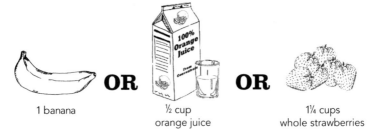

OR

OR

1 banana

½ cup
orange juice

1¼ cups
whole strawberries

If you have more than one serving at a meal, you can choose different types of fruit or have two servings of one fruit.

What are healthy ways to eat fruit?

■ Eat fruits raw or cooked, as juice with no sugar added, canned in their own juice, or dried.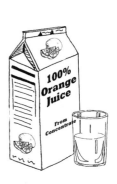

■ Buy smaller pieces of fruit.

■ Eat pieces of fruit rather than drinking fruit juice. Pieces of fruit are more filling.

■ Drink fruit juice in small amounts.

■ Save high-sugar and high-fat fruit desserts such as peach cobbler or cherry pie for special occasions.

Milk and yogurt

Milk and yogurt give you energy, protein, fat, calcium, vitamin A, and other vitamins and minerals.

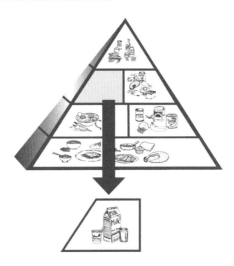

How much is a serving of milk and yogurt?
Examples of 1 serving:

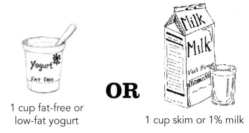

1 cup fat-free or
low-fat yogurt

OR

1 cup skim or 1% milk

Note: If you are pregnant or breastfeeding, have four to five servings of milk and yogurt each day.

What are healthy ways to have milk and yogurt?

- Drink fat-free (skim or nonfat) or low-fat (1%) milk.
- Eat low-fat or fat-free fruit yogurt sweetened with a low-calorie sweetener.
- Use low-fat plain yogurt as a substitute for sour cream.

Meat and meat substitutes

The meat and meat substitutes group includes meat, poultry, eggs, cheese, fish, and tofu. Eat small amounts of some of these foods each day.

Meat and meat substitutes help your body build tissue and muscles. They also give your body energy and vitamins and minerals.

Examples of meat and meat substitutes include

- chicken
- fish
- beef

- eggs
- peanut butter
- tofu

- cheese
- ham
- pork

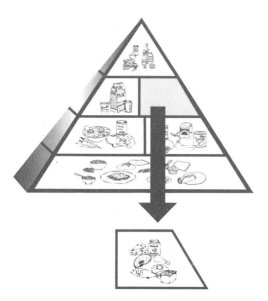

How much is a serving of meat or meat substitute?

Examples of 1 serving:

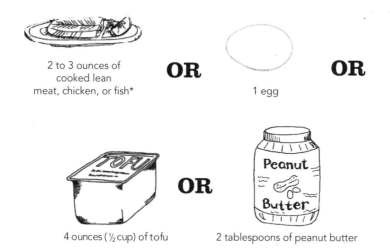

2 to 3 ounces of
cooked lean
meat, chicken, or fish*

OR

1 egg

OR

4 ounces (½ cup) of tofu

OR

2 tablespoons of peanut butter

Note: Two to three ounces of meat (after cooking) is about the size of a deck of cards.

What are healthy ways to eat meat or meat substitutes?

- Buy cuts of beef, pork, ham, and lamb that have only a little fat on them. Trim off extra fat.

- Eat chicken or turkey without the skin.

- Cook meat or meat substitutes in low-fat ways:
  - broil
  - steam
  - grill
  - roast
  - stew
  - stir-fry

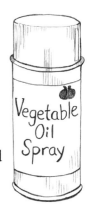

- Cook eggs with a small amount of fat or use cooking spray.

- Limit the amounts of nuts, peanut butter, and fried chicken that you eat. They are high in fat.

- Choose low-fat or fat-free cheese.

Fats and sweets

Limit the amounts of fats and sweets you eat. They have calories, but not much nutrition. Some contain saturated fats and cholesterol that increase your risk of heart disease. Limiting these foods will help you lose weight and keep your blood glucose and blood fats under control.

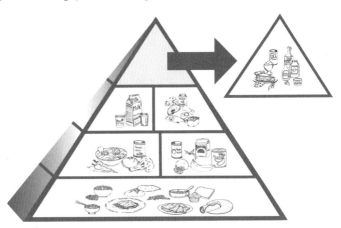

Examples of fats include
- salad dressing
- oil
- butter
- margarine
- avocado
- olives

Examples of sweets include
- regular soda
- ice cream
- cake
- cookies
- pie
- candy

How much is a serving of sweets?
Examples of 1 serving:

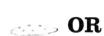 **OR** **OR** **OR**

1 3-inch cookie   1 plain cake doughnut   4 chocolate kisses   1 tablespoon maple syrup

How much is a serving of fat?
Examples of 1 serving:

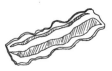 **OR**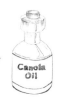

1 strip of bacon   1 teaspoon of oil

Examples of 2 servings:

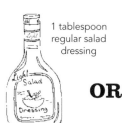

1 tablespoon regular salad dressing

OR

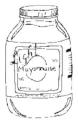

2 tablespoons light salad dressing **PLUS** 1 tablespoon light mayonaise

How can I satisfy my sweet tooth?

It's okay to have sweets once in a while. Try having sugar-free popsicles, diet soda, fat-free ice cream or frozen yogurt, or sugar-free hot cocoa mix.

Other tips:

- Share desserts in restaurants.
- Order small or child-size servings of ice cream or frozen yogurt.
- Divide homemade desserts into small servings and wrap each individually. Freeze extra servings.
- Don't keep dishes of candy in the house or at work.

Remember, fat-free and low-sugar foods still have calories. Talk with your diabetes teacher about how to fit sweets into your meal plan.

Alcohol

Alcohol has calories but no nutrients. If you drink alcohol on an empty stomach, it can make your blood glucose level too low. Alcohol also can raise your blood fats. If you want to drink alcohol, talk with your doctor or diabetes teacher about how it fits into your meal plan.

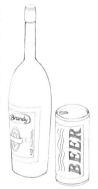

Your meal plan

Plan your meals and snacks for one day.
(Work with your diabetes teacher if you need help.)

Breakfast

Food Group	Food	How Much
_____	_____	_____
_____	_____	_____
_____	_____	_____
_____	_____	_____
_____	_____	_____
_____	_____	_____

Snack

Food Group	Food	How Much
_____	_____	_____
_____	_____	_____
_____	_____	_____

Lunch

Food Group	Food	How Much
_____	_____	_____
_____	_____	_____
_____	_____	_____
_____	_____	_____
_____	_____	_____

Snack

Food Group	Food	How Much
_____	_____	_____
_____	_____	_____
_____	_____	_____

Dinner	Food Group	Food	How Much
	_____	_____	_____
	_____	_____	_____
	_____	_____	_____
	_____	_____	_____
	_____	_____	_____

Snack	Food Group	Food	How Much
	_____	_____	_____
	_____	_____	_____
	_____	_____	_____

Measuring your food

To make sure your food servings are the right size, use measuring cups, measuring spoons, and a food scale. Also, the Nutrition Facts label on food packages tells you how much of that food is in one serving.

These tips will help you choose the right serving sizes:

- Measure a serving size of dry cereal or hot cereal, pasta, or rice and pour it into a bowl or plate. The next time you eat that food, use the same bowl or plate and fill it to the same level.

- For one serving of milk, measure 1 cup and pour it into a glass. See how high it fills the glass. Always drink milk out of that size glass.

- Meat weighs more before it's cooked. For example, 4 ounces of raw meat will weigh about 3 ounces after cooking. For meat with a bone, like a pork chop or chicken leg, cook 5 ounces raw to get 3 ounces cooked.

- One serving of meat or meat substitute is about the size and thickness of the palm of your hand or a deck of cards.

- A small fist is equal to about ½ cup of fruit, vegetables, or starches like rice.

- A small fist is equal to 1 small piece of fresh fruit.

- A thumb is equal to about 1 ounce of meat or cheese.

- The tip of a thumb is equal to about 1 teaspoon.

When you are sick

It's important to take care of your diabetes even when you're ill. Here are some tips on what to do:

- Even if you can't keep food down, keep taking your diabetes medicine.

- Drink at least one cup (8 ounces) of water or other calorie-free, caffeine-free liquid every hour while you're awake.

- If you can't eat your usual food, try drinking juice or eating crackers, popsicles, or soup.

- If you can't eat at all, drink clear liquids such as ginger ale. Eat or drink something with sugar in it if you have trouble keeping food down, because you still need calories. If you don't have enough calories, you increase your risk of hypoglycemia (low blood sugar).

- Make sure that you check your blood glucose. Your blood glucose level may be high even if you're not eating.

- Call your doctor right away if you throw up more than once or have diarrhea for more than six hours.

Points to remember

- What, when, and how much you eat all affect your blood glucose level.

- You can keep your blood glucose at a healthy level if you
  - Eat about the same amount of food each day.
  - Eat at about the same times each day.
  - Take your medicines at the same times each day.
  - Exercise at the same times each day.

- Every day, choose foods from these food groups: starches, vegetables, fruit, meat and meat substitutes, and milk and yogurt. How much of each depends on how many calories you need a day.

- Limit the amounts of fats and sweets you eat each day.

How to find more help

Diabetes Teachers (nurses, dietitians, pharmacists, and other health professionals)

- To find a diabetes teacher near you, call the American Association of Diabetes Educators toll-free at 1-800-TEAMUP4 (1-800-832-6874) or see *www.diabeteseducator.org* and click on "Find A Diabetes Educator."

Recognized Diabetes Education Programs
(teaching programs approved by the American Diabetes Association)

- To find a program near you, call toll-free 1-800-DIABETES (1-800-342-2383) or see *www.diabetes.org/education/edustate2.asp?loc=x.*

Dietitians

- To find a dietitian near you, call the American Dietetic Association's National Center for Nutrition and Dietetics toll-free at 1-800-366-1655 or see *www.eatright.org* and click on "Find a Nutrition Professional."

Delicious Drinks

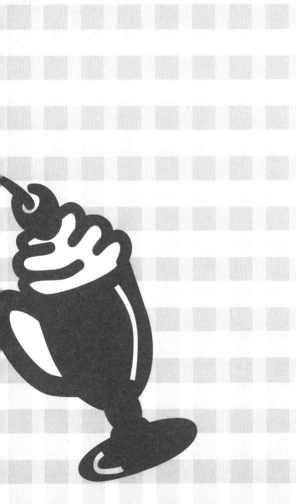

Cherry Freeze

At our local ice cream parlor they have a drink they call a "Freeze," which is a combination of a slushy and ice cream blended together. I love it! However, as usual, it is way too high in calories and sugars for me to enjoy on a regular basis. I created my own version and it is absolutely fantastic!

1	(0.3-ounce) box sugar-free cherry gelatin mix (do not make as directed on box)	1/2 cup cold water
1/2	cup boiling water	2 cups low-fat frozen vanilla yogurt
20	ice cubes	1 teaspoon vanilla extract

- Dissolve the gelatin in the boiling water.
- Pour the gelatin into a blender and add the ice cubes and cold water. Pulse until well blended. Stir in between pulses to mix the ingredients together. (Remember when making this drink that patience is a virtue. It takes time, but the end result is well worth the patience it takes to make.)
- Add the frozen yogurt and vanilla. Continue pulsing and stirring until completely blended and creamy.
- Serve immediately.

Yield: 4 (1-cup) servings

Calories: 62 (23% fat); Total Fat: 2 gm; Cholesterol: 5 mg; Carbohydrate: 7 gm; Dietary Fiber: 0 gm; Protein: 4 gm; Sodium: 105 mg
Diabetic Exchanges: $1/2$ other carbohydrate, $1/2$ fat

Preparation time: 15 minutes or less

Menu Idea: This is terrific for lunch with the Hens & Eggs Tossed Salad on page 145 in this book.

Frozen Chocolate Mocha

I was so thrilled with my results when I came up with this drink. It tastes so fattening, but it's not. Life is so good!

1 teaspoon unsweetened cocoa powder	1/2 cup brewed coffee, at room temperature or chilled
3 individual packets Splenda	1/3 cup low-fat frozen vanilla yogurt
4 ice cubes	

- Combine the cocoa powder, Splenda, ice cubes, coffee, and frozen yogurt in a blender.
- Cover and process on the highest speed for 1 to 2 minutes or until the ice is completely crushed and the drink is blended.
- Pour into a pretty glass.

Yield: 1 (1-cup) serving

Calories: 55; Total Fat: 1 gm; Percent Fat Calories: 19%; Cholesterol: 3 mg; Carbohydrate: 9 gm; Dietary Fiber: 0 gm; Protein: 3 gm; Sodium: 32 mg
Diabetic Exchanges: 1/2 other carbohydrate

 Preparation time: 3 minutes or less

Frozen Mocha:

Follow the Frozen Chocolate Mocha recipe, but use only 2 packets of Splenda and eliminate the cocoa powder.

Calories: 44 (20% fat); Total Fat: 1 gm; Cholesterol: 3 mg; Carbohydrate: 7 gm; Dietary Fiber: 0 gm; Protein: 2 gm; Sodium: 32 mg
Diabetic Exchanges: 1/2 other carbohydrate

 Menu Idea: Have Popeye's Favorite Salad (spinach, of course), on page 143 in this book, with this drink for a refreshing lunch.

Very Cherry Protein Drink

I can't stand the high cost or chalky taste of a lot of protein drinks, so I came up with this unique combination. It's got a little "zip" from the lemon-lime soda, creaminess from the puréed cottage cheese, and just the right amount of sweetness from the cherries along with a little extra help from Splenda.

1	cup frozen no-sugar-added dark sweet cherries	8	ice cubes
2	cups sugar-free lemon-lime soda	1	cup fat-free cottage cheese
		4	to 5 individual packets Splenda

- In a blender combine the cherries, soda, ice cubes, cottage cheese, and Splenda. Process on high until the mixture is smooth and creamy.
- Serve immediately.

Yield: 5 (1-cup) servings

Calories: 81 (0% fat); Total Fat: 0 gm; Cholesterol: 2 mg; Carbohydrate: 14 gm; Dietary Fiber: 1 gm; Protein: 6 gm; Sodium: 167 mg
Diabetic Exchanges: 1 fruit, 1 very lean meat

Preparation time: 5 minutes or less

Menu Idea: This is a breakfast in itself packed with loads of healthy nutrition to keep you going.

Peaches & Cream Smoothie

Oh my gosh! This is so fantastic! It's hard to believe it's low in sugar and calories. I can only hope that drinks in heaven will taste this good.

¼ cup Splenda Granular	1 (11-ounce) can mandarin oranges in light syrup, undrained
18 ice cubes	
2 cups low-fat frozen vanilla yogurt	1 (8¼-ounce) can sliced light peaches in pear juice and water, undrained
1 teaspoon vanilla extract	

- In a blender or smoothie machine combine the Splenda, ice cubes, frozen yogurt, vanilla, mandarin oranges with juice, and peaches with juice. Process, covered, on the highest speed until smooth and creamy.
- You may need to turn the blender off occasionally and stir with a long spoon or spatula if the ingredients do not blend together at first.

Yield: 5 (1-cup) servings

Calories: 110 (10% fat); Total Fat: 1 gm; Cholesterol: 4 mg; Carbohydrate: 22 gm; Dietary Fiber: 0 gm; Protein: 2 gm; Sodium: 45 mg
Diabetic Exchanges: 1 fruit, 1 other carbohydrate

Preparation time: 5 minutes or less

Menu Idea: If you want everyone to think you're a goddess in the kitchen, serve this! For a refreshing "pick-me-up" on hot days serve alone or with a fresh vegetable tray.

Virgin Fuzzy Navel Slushy

This nonalcoholic slushy tastes like peaches and oranges mixed together and is out-of-this-world terrific!

I	(11-ounce) can mandarin oranges in light syrup, undrained	2	tablespoons Splenda Granular
I	(8¹/4-ounce) can sliced lite peaches in pear juice and water, undrained	18	ice cubes

- In a blender or smoothie machine combine the mandarin oranges with juice, peaches with juice, and Splenda. Add the ice cubes.
- Put the lid on the blender and process on high speed until slushy.

Yield: 4 (1-cup) servings

Calories: 81 (0% fat); Total Fat: 0 gm; Cholesterol: 0 mg; Carbohydrate: 19 gm;
Dietary Fiber: 1 gm; Protein: 0 gm; Sodium: 11 mg
Diabetic Exchanges: 1¹/2 fruit

Preparation time: 5 minutes or less

Menu Idea: This fun, fruity slushy tastes great with salads or sandwiches.

Slushy

What child doesn't like a cold slushy to drink on a hot day? This homemade slushy is the answer to giving them what they want without the high cost of going to the local ice cream parlor and also without the high sugar content.

10 plus 10 ice cubes 1/2 cup cold water 1/2 cup boiling water	1 (0.3-ounce) box of your favorite flavor sugar-free gelatin mix (do not make as directed on box)

- Combine 10 ice cubes and the cold water in a blender.
- Stir the gelatin into the boiling water and keep stirring until completely dissolved.
- Put the lid on the blender and process on high for about 1 minute. You may have to stop the blender occasionally to stir with a spoon if the mixture stops blending.
- Remove the lid and slowly add the hot gelatin while processing on low speed.
- Add 10 more ice cubes. Put the lid back on the blender and process until there are no more chunks of ice and the drink is slushy.
- Pour into glasses. Drink immediately.

Yield: 3 (1-cup) servings

Calories: 9 (0% fat); Total Fat: 0 gm; Cholesterol: 0 mg; Carbohydrate: 0 gm;
Dietary Fiber: 0 gm; Protein: 2 gm; Sodium: 67 mg
Diabetic Exchanges: Free

Preparation time: 10 minutes or less

Menu Ideas: This fun drink is good by itself for a snack or with lunch-time favorites such as Bacon, Lettuce, and Tomato Salad (page 96) from *Busy People's Low-Fat Cookbook* or the Kickin' Chicken Spread on page 112 in this book.

Tropical Mango Smoothie

This thick, cold, refreshing, and filling drink reminds me of the tropical islands. The good news is that it's low in sugar and will help you keep that healthy shape to wear your swimsuit on the island beaches.

1 (20-ounce) can pineapple chunks in natural juice	1 teaspoon coconut flavoring (found near vanilla extract)
1 cup cubed fresh mango	1 teaspoon banana flavoring (found near vanilla extract)
17 ice cubes	
1/2 cup Splenda Granular	

- Discard 1 cup of juice from the can of pineapple.
- Combine the mango, pineapple, pineapple juice, ice cubes, Splenda, coconut flavoring, and banana flavoring in a blender.
- Process on the highest speed for 1 minute or until all the ingredients are well blended and the ice is completely crushed. Pour into glasses and serve immediately.

Yield: 4 (1-cup) servings

Calories: 94 (0% fat); Total Fat: 0 gm; Cholesterol: 0 mg; Carbohydrate: 22 gm; Dietary Fiber: 1 gm; Protein: 0 gm; Sodium: 8 mg
Diabetic Exchanges: $1\frac{1}{2}$ fruit

Preparation time: 8 minutes or less

Menu Idea: This smoothie is so nutritious and filling that my children and I drank it as a midday snack after they got home from school. It is even satisfying enough to have for breakfast on the run; however, if you want some protein with your breakfast, cook a quick batch of scrambled eggs made with Egg Beaters.

Very Berry Frozen Drink

This berry frozen drink is berry good! Although it's berry bad, I hope my dry humor brought a smile to your face. Oh yes, and I do hope you have a berry good day. Okay, okay! I'll stop!

6 ice cubes	$1/2$ cup low-fat frozen vanilla yogurt
$1\,1/4$ cups frozen mixed berries	
1 cup diet red raspberry soda (I use Diet Rite)	$1/2$ cup fat-free whipped topping (I use Cool Whip Free)
$1/4$ cup fat-free half-and-half	3 tablespoons Splenda Granular

- In a blender, combine the ice cubes, frozen berries, soda, half-and-half, frozen yogurt, whipped topping, and Splenda.
- Process on the highest speed for about 1 minute or until all the ingredients are well blended.

Yield: $2\frac{1}{2}$ (1-cup) servings

Calories: 107 (7% fat); Total Fat: 1 gm; Cholesterol: 2 mg; Carbohydrate: 22 gm; Dietary Fiber: 2 gm; Protein: 3 gm; Sodium: 63 mg
Diabetic Exchanges: 1 fruit, 1 other carbohydrate

Preparation time: 5 minutes or less

Menu Idea: Serve this frozen drink on hot days with a refreshing salad such as the Shrimp Sunshine Salad (page 57) from *Busy People's Down-Home Cooking Without the Down-Home Fat* for a meal that will pick your spirits up and make you feel good inside.

Banana Cream Smoothie

This is so smooth, creamy, and delicious that you may have a difficult time limiting yourself to just one serving. It's definitely a special treat.

1 cup cold water	1 cup skim milk
1 (0.9-ounce) box sugar-free, fat-free banana cream instant pudding mix (do not make as directed on box)	1 cup low-fat frozen vanilla yogurt
	$^1/_4$ cup Splenda Granular
	1 teaspoon vanilla extract
20 ice cubes	

- In a blender, combine the water with the pudding mix. Blend on high for 20 seconds or until the pudding is completely dissolved.
- Add the ice cubes, milk, frozen yogurt, Splenda, and vanilla to the blender and cover.
- Process on high speed. If needed, pulse the blender off and on, stirring in between pulses to make sure all the ice cubes are crushed and the ingredients are blended.
- Once the ingredients are well blended, blend 30 seconds longer to assure a thick, smooth drink.
- Pour into cups or glasses and drink immediately.

Yield: $4^1/_2$ (1-cup) servings

Calories: 80 (0% fat); Total Fat: 0 gm; Cholesterol: 1 mg; Carbohydrate: 16 gm; Dietary Fiber: 0 gm; Protein: 3 gm; Sodium: 282 mg
Diabetic Exchanges: 1 other carbohydrate

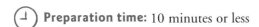 **Preparation time:** 10 minutes or less

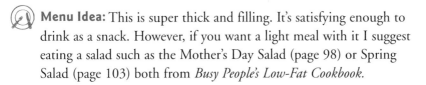 **Menu Idea:** This is super thick and filling. It's satisfying enough to drink as a snack. However, if you want a light meal with it I suggest eating a salad such as the Mother's Day Salad (page 98) or Spring Salad (page 103) both from *Busy People's Low-Fat Cookbook*.

Frozen Raspberry Colada

No doubt about it! You will like this frozen drink from the first sip to the last. Raspberries, pineapple, and coconut are blended together with ice for a winning flavor! (My daughter Ashley named this drink because she says it tastes like a virgin piña colada with raspberries.)

1 (12-ounce) bag frozen red raspberries	1/2 cup Splenda Granular
2 teaspoons coconut extract	1/2 cup diet cherry 7-Up
1 1/2 cups crushed pineapple in pineapple juice, undrained	25 ice cubes, divided

- In a blender or smoothie machine, combine the raspberries, coconut extract, pineapple with juice, Splenda, soda, and 5 ice cubes.
- Cover the blender and process on high speed until the ice turns slushy.
- Stir, bringing the contents from the bottom of the blender to the top. Add 5 more ice cubes.
- Cover the blender and process on high speed until the ice turns slushy.
- Add the remaining ice cubes, 5 at a time, and continue to blend and stir.

Note: You can substitute frozen strawberries for the raspberries to make a frozen strawberry colada.

Yield: 5 (1-cup) servings

(with raspberries) Calories: 101 (0% fat); Total Fat: 0 gm; Cholesterol: 0 mg; Carbohydrate: 24 gm; Dietary Fiber: 3 gm; Protein: 1 gm; Sodium: 10 mg
Diabetic Exchanges: 1 1/2 fruit
(with strawberries) Calories: 80 (0% fat); Total Fat: 0 gm; Cholesterol: 0 mg; Carbohydrate: 19 gm; Dietary Fiber: 2 gm; Protein: 0 gm; Sodium: 11 mg
Diabetic Exchanges: 1 1/2 fruit

🕐 **Preparation time:** 10 minutes or less

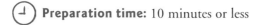 **Menu Idea:** This thick drink is especially refreshing on hot days with Mother's Day Salad (page 98) from *Busy People's Low-Fat Cookbook* and the orange roughy recipe on page 182 in this book.

Apricot Freeze

This frozen beverage is a great alternative for people who don't like to eat their daily recommended amounts of fruit. Now they can drink them instead!

1/2 cup Splenda Granular	1 (15-ounce) can apricot halves in pear juice, undrained
1 cup low-fat frozen vanilla yogurt	1/2 cup sugar-free lemon-lime soda
1 tablespoon unsweetened peach-mango flavoring (found in the tea aisle)	24 ice cubes

- In a blender or smoothie machine, combine the Splenda, frozen yogurt, peach-mango flavoring, apricots with juice, and soda. Add the ice cubes. Process, covered, on the highest speed until smooth and creamy.

Yield: 4 (1-cup) servings

Calories: 88 (8% fat); Total Fat: 1 gm; Cholesterol: 3 mg; Carbohydrate: 20 gm; Dietary Fiber: 2 gm; Protein: 2 gm; Sodium: 31 mg
Diabetic Exchanges: 1 fruit, 1/2 other carbohydrate

Preparation time: 5 minutes or less

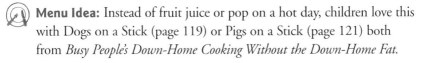 **Menu Idea:** Instead of fruit juice or pop on a hot day, children love this with Dogs on a Stick (page 119) or Pigs on a Stick (page 121) both from *Busy People's Down-Home Cooking Without the Down-Home Fat.*

Super Fruity Strawberry Milk Shakes

The intense fruity flavor is what gives this winning milk shake its name. This drink will definitely add an explosion of fun flavor to any boring day. It's a real hit with the children.

1 **(0.3-ounce) box sugar-free strawberry gelatin, dry (do not make as directed on box)**	**Fat-free whipped cream from a can**
1 **cup boiling water***	5 **fresh large strawberries**
4 **cups low-fat vanilla frozen yogurt, softened (I use Flavorite)**	

- In a medium bowl stir the gelatin into the boiling water until completely dissolved. (If it is not completely dissolved when you combine it with the frozen yogurt you will get clumps.)
- In a large blender or smoothie maker, combine the frozen yogurt and hot gelatin. Process on high for 1 to 2 minutes or until smooth and creamy.
- Pour into glasses.
- Top each serving with a little whipped cream.
- Garnish by cutting a diagonal slit into each strawberry. Place a strawberry on the rim of each glass.
- Serve immediately with a straw, if desired.

*Note: To boil the water quickly, heat it in the microwave for 1 minute.

Yield: 5 (1-cup) servings

Calories: 99 (22% fat); Total Fat: 3 gm; Cholesterol: 8 mg; Carbohydrate: 14 gm; Dietary Fiber: 0 gm; Protein: 6 gm; Sodium: 114 mg
Diabetic Exchanges: 1 other carbohydrate, $\frac{1}{2}$ fat

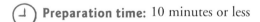 **Preparation time:** 10 minutes or less

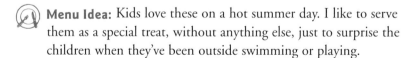 **Menu Idea:** Kids love these on a hot summer day. I like to serve them as a special treat, without anything else, just to surprise the children when they've been outside swimming or playing.

Spiced Chai Tea

I loved the flavor of spiced chai from a local coffeehouse, but when I found out how many calories it had I almost flipped! So I created this scrumptious specialty, which I treat myself to when I want to soothe away a stressful day. It's wonderful!

1 cup water	plus 1 dash pumpkin pie spice
1 chai tea bag	Fat-free whipped cream from a can
2 tablespoons fat-free half-and-half	
2 individual packets Splenda	

- Heat the water in a mug in the microwave for 1 minute and 20 seconds.
- Remove the water from the microwave and place the chai tea bag in the water. Place a teaspoon on top of the tea bag to keep it immersed in the water. Let it steep for 2 minutes. Remove the tea bag.
- Stir in the half-and-half, Splenda, and 1 dash of pumpkin pie spice, stirring until the Splenda and pumpkin pie spice are dissolved.
- Microwave for 30 seconds.
- Top with the whipped cream. Sprinkle lightly with the remaining dash of pumpkin pie spice, if desired.

Yield: 1 (1-cup) serving

Calories: 44 (0% fat); Total Fat: 0 gm; Cholesterol: 0 mg; Carbohydrate: 9 gm;
Dietary Fiber: 0 gm; Protein: 2 gm; Sodium: 35 mg
Diabetic Exchanges: $\frac{1}{2}$ other carbohydrate

Preparation time: 5 minutes or less

Menu Idea: This is a perfect dessert drink all by itself after any meal. A couple Spice Cookies (only 5 carbs), on page 219 in *Busy People's Low-Fat Cookbook*, is a flavorful accompaniment.

Hot Chocolate—Skinny Style

Never miss high-calorie hot chocolate again!

1 cup skim milk	1 tablespoon Splenda Granular
1 tablespoon unsweetened cocoa powder	

- Combine the milk and cocoa powder in a blender. Cover and blend on high for 10 seconds or until well blended.
- Pour into a coffee cup or small mug.
- Microwave for 1 minute or until completely heated.
- Stir in the Splenda until completely dissolved and well blended. If a sweeter taste is preferred add more Splenda, 1 teaspoon at a time.
- Serve hot.

Note: For numerous servings simply multiply the above recipe by the number of servings you need. And for variations you can add different flavorings with the Splenda. Try 1 or 2 drops of mint, 1 tablespoon sugar-free vanilla syrup, or 1 tablespoon sugar-free hazelnut syrup. The nutritional information is the same with the different flavors.

Yield: 1 (1-cup) serving

Calories: 113 (8% fat); Total Fat: 1 gm; Cholesterol: 5 mg; Carbohydrate: 17 gm; Dietary Fiber: 1 gm; Protein: 9 gm; Sodium: 127 mg
Diabetic Exchanges: 1 skim milk

Preparation time: 3 minutes or less

Menu Idea: For a low-calorie chocolate overload have this with Chocolate Mint Cookie Squares on page 252 of this book.

Mocha Hot Chocolate—Skinny Style

You'll never want to pay the high price at coffeehouses for this special coffee drink again!

1	cup skim milk	1	tablespoon unsweetened cocoa powder
1	teaspoon instant coffee granules	1	tablespoon Splenda Granular

- Combine the milk, instant coffee, and cocoa powder in a blender. Cover and blend on high for 10 seconds or until well blended.
- Pour into a coffee cup or small mug.
- Microwave for 1 minute or until completely heated.
- Stir in the Splenda until completely dissolved and well blended. If a sweeter taste is preferred add more Splenda, 1 teaspoon at a time.
- Serve hot.

Note: See note on opposite page.

Yield: 1 (1-cup) serving

Calories: 115 (8% fat); Total Fat: 1 gm; Cholesterol: 5 mg; Carbohydrate: 17 gm; Dietary Fiber: 1 gm; Protein: 10 gm; Sodium: 128 mg
Diabetic Exchanges: 1 skim milk

Preparation time: 3 minutes or less

Menu Idea: Crunchy Chocolate Kisses (Cookies) on page 248 in this book go great with this drink.

Mint Steamer

This hot caffeine-free mint beverage is the perfect answer to help you relax if you cannot sleep. Old-fashioned home remedies recommended drinking warm milk. With this little bit of flavoring you are going to want to drink this even if you sleep like a baby.

1 cup skim milk	$1/2$ teaspoon vanilla extract
1 $1/2$ teaspoons crème de menthe syrup (found with the ice cream syrups)	1 individual packet Splenda

- Microwave the milk for 1 minute and 20 seconds or until steaming hot.
- Combine the hot milk, syrup, vanilla extract, and Splenda in a blender.
- Put the lid on the blender, but keep the corner of the lid facing away from you slighty opened so the heat from the milk can escape. Otherwise, pressure can build up and the lid could explode off!
- Process on the highest speed for 10 to 20 seconds.
- Pour into a mug.

Yield: 1 serving

Calories: 117 (0% fat); Total Fat: 0 gm; Cholesterol: 5 mg; Carbohydrate: 18 gm; Dietary Fiber: 0 gm; Protein: 8 gm; Sodium: 128 mg
Diabetic Exchanges: 1 skim milk

Preparation time: 3 minutes or less

Menu Idea: The light green color makes this a perfect caffeine-free, alcohol-free hot beverage to serve in celebration of St. Patrick's Day. Its smooth mint and vanilla flavor complements and enhances Brownie Cookies (page 217) from *Busy People's Low-Fat Cookbook*.

Vanilla Steamer

I love the flavor of steamers at coffeehouses, but I didn't want the hassle of buying a cappuccino machine. So I came up with these fantastic and absolutely delicious homemade steamers that are every bit as wonderful and foamy on top as those at the expensive specialty coffee shops.

1 cup skim milk	1 tablespoon sugar-free vanilla syrup
1 to 2 individual packets Splenda (depending on how sweet you like it)	

- Heat the milk in the microwave for 1 minute and 20 seconds or until piping hot.
- Pour the hot milk into a blender.
- Add the Splenda and vanilla syrup.
- Put the lid on the blender, but keep the corner of the lid facing away from you slightly opened so the heat from the milk can escape. Otherwise, pressure can build up and the lid could explode off!
- Process on the highest speed for about 10 seconds or until the milk is foamy.
- Pour into a mug.

Note: Use sugar-free hazelnut syrup or a dash of pumpkin spice instead of the vanilla syrup for a different flavor. The nutritional information stays the same.

Yield: 1 serving

Calories: 90 (0% fat); Total Fat: 0 gm; Cholesterol: 5 mg; Carbohydrate: 13 gm; Dietary Fiber: 0 gm; Protein: 8 gm; Sodium: 127 mg
Diabetic Exchanges: 1 skim milk

Preparation time: 3 minutes or less

Menu Idea: This is great to sip on at the end of a long day to help soothe you into a comfy mood. It is so special it can be served instead of traditional coffee for fancy meals or breakfasts. Serve with my assorted low-fat cookies from *Busy People's Low-Fat Cookbook,* such as Brownie Cookies on page 217, Apple Oatmeal Cookies on page 232, or Chocolate Pecan Cookies on page 227.

Café Latte

You may never want to pay the high price of coffeehouse café lattes again when you realize how fast, easy, and inexpensively these can be made at home, and with almost no fat.

1 **cup skim milk**	1 **teaspoon instant coffee granules**

- Heat the milk in the microwave for 1 minute and 20 seconds or until piping hot.
- Combine the hot milk and instant coffee in a blender.
- Put the lid on the blender, but keep the corner of the lid facing away from you slightly opened so the heat from the milk can escape. Otherwise, pressure can build up and the lid could explode off!
- Process on high for 10 to 20 seconds.
- Pour into a mug.

Yield: 1 serving

Calories: 101 (10% fat); Total Fat: 1 gm; Cholesterol: 5 mg; Carbohydrate: 14 gm; Dietary Fiber: 0 gm; Protein: 9 gm; Sodium: 141 mg
Diabetic Exchanges: 1 skim milk

Preparation time: 3 minutes or less

Menu Idea: For an impressive presentation serve this instead of traditional coffee with beautiful desserts like Pumpkin Cake (page 202) or Almond Cake (page 194) which are both from *Busy People's Slow Cooker Cookbook.*

Mocha Café Latte

This blends the flavors of hot chocolate and coffee together perfectly, like a match made in heaven!

1 **cup skim milk**	1 **teaspoon unsweetened cocoa powder**
1 **teaspoon instant coffee granules**	1 **individual packet Splenda**
1 **tablespoon sugar-free vanilla syrup (I use Davinci Gourmet, found in coffee and tea aisle)**	1 **tablespoon fat-free whipped topping (I use Cool Whip)**

- Heat the milk in the microwave for 1 minute and 20 seconds or until piping hot.
- Pour the hot milk into a blender.
- Add the instant coffee, vanilla syrup, cocoa powder, and Splenda.
- Put the lid on the blender, but keep the corner of the lid facing away from you slightly opened so the heat from the milk can escape. Otherwise, pressure can build up and the lid could explode off!
- Process on high for 10 to 20 seconds.
- Pour into a mug.
- Top with the whipped topping. If desired, sprinkle the whipped topping very lightly with cocoa powder.

Yield: 1 serving

Calories: 119 (10% fat); Total Fat: 1 gm; Cholesterol: 5 mg; Carbohydrate: 18 gm; Dietary Fiber: 0 gm; Protein: 9 gm; Sodium: 144 mg
Diabetic Exchanges: 1 skim milk

Preparation time: 3 minutes or less

Menu Idea: *Busy People's Slow Cooker Cookbook* has a Black Forest Upside-Down Cake (page 208) that tastes out of this world with this hot beverage! However, this beverage is so wonderful just the way it is: hot, smooth, and oh-so creamy and chocolaty, that nothing else is needed. It satisfies like a dessert and a coffee together.

Hot Caramel Cider

Sometimes I even amaze myself with the creative low-calorie, low-sugar and fat-free beverages I've created for this book. This cider is one of them. If you like caramel apples and hot cider you are going to love this. It's fabulous!

1 cup water	1/2 tablespoon fat-free caramel syrup
1 (0.14-ounce) envelope instant sugar-free low-calorie spiced cider drink mix, dry (do not make as directed on the box)	1 tablespoon fat-free whipped topping (I use Cool Whip)

- Microwave the water in a coffee mug for 1 minute.
- Stir in the spiced cider mix until completely dissolved.
- Stir three-fourths of the caramel into the hot cider. Stir until completely dissolved.
- Top with whipped dessert topping.
- Drizzle the remaining caramel over the whipped topping.
- Drink immediately.

Yield: 1 (1-cup) serving

Calories: 55 (0% fat); Total Fat: 0 gm; Cholesterol: 0 mg; Carbohydrate: 13 gm; Dietary Fiber: 0 gm; Protein: 0 gm; Sodium: 60 mg
Diabetic Exchanges: 1 other carbohydrate

Preparation time: 2 minutes or less

 Menu Idea: To curb a sweet tooth this will do the trick by itself. However, if you want something to sink your teeth into, serve this beverage with some terrific Cranberry or Raisin Oatmeal Cookies (page 148) from *Busy People's Down-Home Cooking Without the Down-Home Fat.*

Butter Rum Spiced Cider

The aroma of this hot beverage has a medicinal and soothing effect. It is especially comforting when you feel achy.

1 cup water	1/2 teaspoon imitation rum flavoring (in the spice section of store near vanilla)
1 (0.14-ounce) envelope instant sugar-free low-calorie spiced cider drink mix, dry (do not make as directed on the box)	1/2 teaspoon butter flavoring (in spice section of store near vanilla)

- Microwave the water in a coffee mug for 1 minute or until very hot.
- Stir in the spiced cider mix until completely dissolved.
- Stir the rum and butter flavorings into the hot cider until completely dissolved.
- Drink immediately.

Yield: 1 (1-cup) serving

Calories: 28 (0% fat); Total Fat: 0 gm; Cholesterol: 0 mg; Carbohydrate: 5 gm; Dietary Fiber: 0 gm; Protein: 0 gm; Sodium: 30 mg
Diabetic Exchanges: 1/2 other carbohydrate

Preparation time: 2 minutes or less

Menu Idea: If you are not feeling well, for an old-fashioned home remedy, drink this while eating a bowl of hot chicken noodle soup. I also like this with Molasses Cookies (page 134) from *Busy People's Down-Home Cooking Without the Down-Home Fat.*

Red Hot Chocolate

The flavors of creamy chocolate and spicy red-hot candies make for a special treat you are sure to enjoy!

1 cup water	1/2 tablespoon cinnamon red-hot candies
1 (0.29-ounce) envelope diet hot chocolate mix	

- Microwave the water in a coffee mug for 1 minute or until very hot.
- Stir in the hot chocolate mix and red-hot candies. Stir for about 1 minute or until all the hot chocolate mix and candies are dissolved.
- Drink immediately.

Yield: 1 (1-cup) serving

Calories: 55 (6% fat); Total Fat: trace; Cholesterol: 0 mg; Carbohydrate: 12 gm; Dietary Fiber: 1 gm; Protein: 1 gm; Sodium: 85 mg
Diabetic Exchanges: 1 other carbohydrate

Preparation time: 2 minutes or less

Menu Idea: This slightly spicy hot chocolate tastes great with fat-free popcorn on a cold winter night or after being outside in the snow. Now isn't it nice that we are able to enjoy a sweet and salty snack completely guilt free? To top it off, this snack combination is actually healthy for you too! Life is so good!

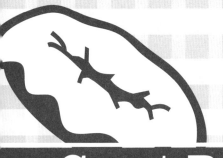

Great Beginnings

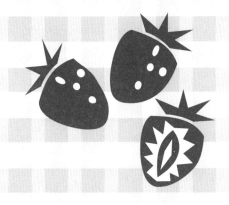

Southwestern Breakfast Casserole

This is a very good vegetarian casserole. My family likes it for brunch served with fat-free sour cream and diced fresh tomatoes.

6 (7-inch) flour tortillas, torn into 2-inch pieces	$^3/_4$ cup liquid egg substitute
1 plus $^1/_2$ cup shredded light four-cheese Mexican cheese (I use Sargento)	2 (4.5-ounce) cans chopped green chilies
1 (12-ounce) can evaporated skim milk	$^1/_2$ cup salsa (mild or spicy)

- Preheat a slow cooker on high. Coat the inside of the slow cooker with nonfat cooking spray.
- In a bowl combine the tortillas, 1 cup cheese, evaporated milk, egg substitute, chilies, and salsa. Mix well and pour into the slow cooker.
- Cover with two layers of paper towels before putting on the lid.
- Cover and cook on high for $3^1/_2$ hours.
- Sprinkle the remaining $^1/_2$ cup cheese on top before serving.

Yield: 4 (1-cup) servings

Calories: 395 (18% fat); Total Fat: 8 gm; Cholesterol: 18 mg; Carbohydrate: 50 gm; Dietary Fiber: 5 gm; Protein: 29 gm; Sodium: 1375 mg
Diabetic Exchanges: 2 starch, 1 skim milk, 1 vegetable, $2^1/_2$ lean meat

Preparation time: 10 minutes or less

Menu Idea: This spicy breakfast casserole tastes good with the Fresh Fruit Salad on page 135 of this book.

Breakfast Scramble

Don't limit this great entrée to breakfast only. It's hearty enough for dinner and great for brunch too.

2 tablespoons fat-free, reduced-sodium chicken broth	1/2 cup chopped frozen onion (or 1/2 medium onion, chopped)
1 pound frozen hash browns	1 cup liquid egg substitute
8 ounces extra-lean honey smoked ham, chopped (from the deli)	1 tablespoon chopped fresh chives
	1 cup shredded fat-free Cheddar cheese (I use Kraft)

- Coat a nonstick 12-inch skillet with nonfat cooking spray.
- Combine the chicken broth, hash browns, ham, and onion in the skillet.
- Cover and cook over medium heat for 10 minutes or until the potatoes are tender, stirring frequently.
- Add the egg substitute and chives. Cook, stirring frequently, until the eggs are fully cooked.
- Remove from the heat and gently stir in the cheese before serving.

Yield: 4 servings

Calories: 246 (13% fat); Total Fat: 4 gm; Cholesterol: 32 mg; Carbohydrate: 24 gm; Dietary Fiber: 2 gm; Protein: 28 gm; Sodium: 1173 mg
Diabetic Exchanges: 3 very lean meat, 1 1/2 starch

Southwestern Breakfast Scramble: Follow the Breakfast Scramble recipe, omitting the chives and onion. Once completely cooked, heat 1 cup of your favorite salsa in the microwave for 1 minute or until fully heated. Pour 1/4 cup salsa over each serving.

Calories: 258 (13% fat); Total Fat: 4 gm; Cholesterol: 32 mg; Carbohydrate: 25 gm; Dietary Fiber: 2 gm; Protein: 28 gm; Sodium: 1452 mg
Diabetic Exchanges: 3 very lean meat, 1 1/2 starch

Italian Breakfast Scramble: Follow the Breakfast Scramble recipe, omitting the chives. Once completely cooked, heat 1 cup of your favorite fat-free spaghetti sauce in the microwave for 1 minute or until fully heated. Pour ¼ cup spaghetti sauce over each serving. (I use Ragú Light pasta sauce.)

Calories: 267 (12% fat); Total Fat: 4 gm; Cholesterol: 32 mg; Carbohydrate: 29 gm;
Dietary Fiber: 3 gm; Protein: 29 gm; Sodium: 1368 mg
Diabetic Exchanges: 3 very lean meat, 1½ starch, 1 vegetable

Preparation time: 10 minutes or less
Cooking time: 10 minutes or less
Total time: 20 minutes or less

Menu Idea: Spiced Chai Tea on page 53 of this book served with a side dish of Portobello Garlic Mushrooms (page 13) from *Busy People's Down-Home Cooking Without the Down-Home Fat* will make this a breakfast they'll remember!

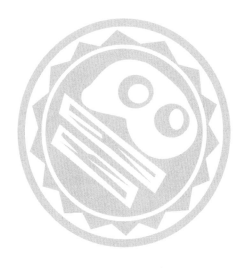

Spinach Scramble

This entrée is an excellent choice when you need a quick meal for breakfast, brunch, lunch, or dinner.

1 ounce extra-lean deli smoked ham (about 1 or 2 slices depending on size), chopped	2 tablespoons fat-free half-and-half
1 cup fresh spinach (about one handful)	1/4 cup fat-free shredded Cheddar cheese
3 egg whites*	1/4 teaspoon garlic salt or salt-free Mrs. Dash (optional)
1 egg	

- Combine the ham and spinach in a 12-inch nonstick skillet over medium heat. (No need to coat the skillet with cooking spray.) Cook, covered, for about 2 minutes or until the spinach leaves are wilted but still tender.
- In a bowl, using a fork or whisk, stir together the egg whites, egg, and half-and-half until well mixed.
- Pour the egg mixture into the skillet with the ham and spinach.
- Using a spatula, scrape the bottom of the skillet constantly, turning over and mixing until the eggs are still lightly wet.
- Sprinkle the cheese on top.
- Cover and cook for 1 minute longer or until the cheese is melted.
- If desired, lightly sprinkle garlic salt or Mrs. Dash seasoning over the dish.
- Serve immediately.

Note: Two-third cup liquid egg substitute can be used in place of egg whites and egg if desired. This will eliminate 4 grams of fat from the total recipe or 2 grams per serving.

Yield: 2 (1-cup) servings

Calories: 117 (25% fat); Total Fat: 3 gm; Cholesterol: 115 mg; Carbohydrate: 5 gm;
Dietary Fiber: 0 gm; Protein: 17 gm; Sodium: 563 mg
Diabetic Exchanges: 1 vegetable, 2$\frac{1}{2}$ very lean meat

Preparation Time: 3 minutes
Cooking time: 10 minutes or less
Total time: 13 minutes or less

Menu Ideas: For lunch or dinner I like serving this with the
Cucumber Dill Salad (page 90) from *Busy People's Low-Fat Cookbook*
and Garlic Crisps (page 29) from *Busy People's Down-Home Cooking
Without the Down-Home Fat.* For breakfast or brunch, Garlic Toast
(page 61) from *Busy People's Low-Fat Cookbook* tastes great with this
along with Peach Tea (page 204) from *Busy People's Down-Home
Cooking Without the Down-Home Fat.*

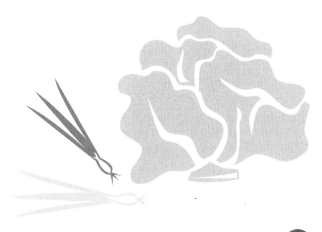

Puffy Herb Omelet with Cheese

This super fluffy and extra light omelet will impress even the most discriminating of guests. Don't be surprised if they think you've studied to be a gourmet chef.

3	egg whites	1/4	teaspoon Mrs. Dash salt-free original seasoning blend
1	tablespoon cold water	1/4	teaspoon garlic salt
1	egg	1/4	cup fat-free shredded Cheddar cheese
1/4	teaspoon lemon pepper seasoning		

- Preheat the oven to 450 degrees.
- In a medium mixing bowl using an electric mixer on high speed, beat together the egg whites and water for 1 to 2 minutes or until stiff peaks form.
- Once the egg whites are beaten, heat a 12-inch ovenproof, nonstick skillet over medium-high heat.
- Add the whole egg, lemon pepper seasoning, Mrs. Dash, and garlic salt to the egg whites. Continue beating on high speed for 1 minute longer.
- Coat the heated skillet with nonfat cooking spray.
- Pour the egg mixture into the skillet and cook for 1 to 2 minutes.
- Put the skillet in the oven for 2 minutes. Remove the skillet and sprinkle the cheese evenly over the omelet. Return the omelet to the oven for 60 to 90 seconds, just long enough to melt the cheese. A sharp knife inserted in the center will come out clean when the omelet is done.
- Remove the omelet from the oven and spray the top of the omelet with nonfat cooking spray. (This prevents the cheese from becoming rubbery or chewy.)

- Let the omelet sit for about 1 minute longer. The internal heat from the omelet will cook any of the egg that is not thoroughly cooked. (Not overcooking the omelet keeps it moist.)
- Fold the omelet in half with a spatula and cut into 2 servings.
- Serve immediately.

Note: This omelet also tastes good with ¾ cup sautéed sliced fresh mushrooms or for a Greek touch substitute feta for the Cheddar and add ½ cup sautéed chopped onion and tomato to the omelet.

Yield: 2 servings

(plain) Calories: 85 (28% fat); Total Fat: 3 gm; Cholesterol: 109 mg; Carbohydrate: 2 gm; Dietary Fiber: 0 gm; Protein: 13 gm; Sodium: 374 mg
Diabetic Exchanges: 2 very lean meat
(with mushrooms) Calories: 91 (26% fat); Total Fat: 3 gm; Cholesterol: 109 mg; Carbohydrate: 3 gm; Dietary Fiber: 0 gm; Protein: 14 gm; Sodium: 375 mg
Diabetic Exchanges: 2 very lean meat
(Greek style) Calories: 107 (23% fat); Total Fat: 3 gm; Cholesterol: 106 mg; Carbohydrate: 8 gm; Dietary Fiber: 1 gm; Protein: 13 gm; Sodium: 579 mg
Diabetic Exchanges: 1½ vegetable, 2 very lean meat

Preparation time: 10 minutes or less
Cooking time: 10 minutes or less
Total time: 20 minutes or less

Menu Idea: This impressive omelet is so light that it can be served with the Fake Bacon recipe (page 30) and the Tropical Passion Fruit Salad (page 89) both from *Busy People's Low-Fat Cookbook.*

Buttermilk Biscuits

My assistant, Brenda Crosser, sent me her version of this recipe while she was in Florida. Her note read: "These are the best buttermilk biscuits ever!" When I retested them for quality assurance I had to agree. They are light and fluffy and melt in your mouth. I like them fresh from the oven best.

2 tablespoons light salad dressing (Miracle Whip)	2 cups reduced-fat baking mix (I use Bisquick)
1 cup low-fat buttermilk	

- Preheat the oven to 350 degrees.
- Coat two baking sheets with nonfat cooking spray. Set aside.
- In a medium mixing bowl, stir together the Miracle Whip, buttermilk, and baking mix until well blended.
- Drop the dough by rounded tablespoonfuls onto the prepared baking sheets. (This is easiest to do by pushing the dough off a measuring tablespoon with the back of another spoon.)
- Bake for 10 to 12 minutes or until the tops of the biscuits are lightly browned.
- Serve fresh from the oven.

Yield: 18 (1-biscuit) servings

Calories: 60 (20% fat); Total Fat: 1 gm; Cholesterol: 1 mg; Carbohydrate: 10 gm; Dietary Fiber: 0 gm; Protein: 2 gm; Sodium: 184 mg
Diabetic Exchanges: $1/2$ starch

Preparation time: 7 minutes or less
Cooking time: 12 minutes or less
Total time: 19 minutes or less

Menu Idea: These are wonderful with soups or stews. These are especially good with Beef Noodle Soup (page 47), with only 12 carbs, or Beef Barley Soup (page 46), with 13 carbs, both from *Busy People's Slow Cooker Cookbook.*

Mushroom Biscuits

This is a step above a traditional biscuit.

1 **(10-count) can refrigerated biscuits (I use Pillsbury)**	1/3 **cup fat-free cottage cheese**
1 **teaspoon minced garlic (I use the kind in a jar)**	1/8 **teaspoon light salt**
	1/4 **cup sliced fresh mushrooms**
1 **teaspoon dried parsley**	2 **tablespoons fat-free Parmesan cheese**

- Preheat the oven to 425 degrees. Coat an 11 x 17-inch jelly roll pan with nonfat cooking spray.
- Arrange the biscuits onto the prepared pan. Set aside.
- In a medium bowl, mix the garlic, parsley, cottage cheese, and salt together with a spoon until smooth and creamy.
- Spread the mixture over the top of each biscuit.
- Top each biscuit with 2 mushroom slices.
- Sprinkle the Parmesan cheese over the mushrooms.
- Bake for 10 minutes.

Yield: 10 (1-biscuit) servings

Calories: 59 (11% fat); Total Fat: 1 gm; Cholesterol: 1 mg; Carbohydrate: 10 gm; Dietary Fiber: 0 gm; Protein: 3 gm; Sodium: 238 mg
Diabetic Exchanges: 1/2 starch

Preparation time: 10 minutes
Cooking time: 10 minutes
Total time: 20 minutes

Menu Ideas: These fancy biscuits will be an asset when dressing up a special meal such as Dilled Chicken and Potatoes (page 135) from *Busy People's Slow Cooker Cookbook*. I suggest having Crunchy Cucumbers with Cream (page 82) from *Busy People's Low-Fat Cookbook* as well.

Bacon Biscuits

The light, smoky flavor of these yummy biscuits is good for breakfast, brunch, or dinner.

2	cups reduced-fat baking mix (I use Bisquick)	2	egg whites
1/2	cup skim milk	I	cup finely shredded fat-free Cheddar cheese (I use Kraft)
1/4	cup applesauce	I	(3-ounce) jar real bacon bits (I use Hormel)

- Preheat the oven to 375 degrees. Coat a baking sheet with nonfat cooking spray.
- In a large bowl, combine the baking mix, milk, applesauce, egg whites, cheese, and bacon bits and mix until well blended.
- Drop by rounded tablespoonfuls onto the prepared baking sheet.
- Bake for 10 to 12 minutes or until golden brown.

Yield: 24 (1-biscuit) servings

Calories: 62 (19% fat); Total Fat: 1 gm; Cholesterol: 3 mg; Carbohydrate: 8 gm; Dietary Fiber: 0 gm; Protein: 4 gm; Sodium: 274 mg
Diabetic Exchanges: 1/2 very lean meat, 1/2 starch

Preparation time: 7 minutes or less
Cooking time: 12 minutes or less
Total time: 19 minutes or less

Menu Ideas: While these smoky flavored biscuits are marvelous at breakfast or brunch, I love them with soup too. Try them with the Steak and Cattlemen's Soup (page 67) or the Chicken Corn Chowder (page 74) both from *Busy People's Low Fat Cookbook.*

Parmesan Biscuits

These are excellent not only with Italian-themed meals but with all home-style meals.

2 tablespoons imitation butter-flavored sprinkles (found in spice or diet section of grocery store)	**½** teaspoon Italian seasoning (found in spice section)
¼ cup finely shredded Parmesan cheese	**l** (l0-count) can refrigerated buttermilk biscuits (I use Pillsbury)

- Preheat the oven to 425 degrees. Coat a baking sheet with nonfat cooking spray.
- Combine the butter-flavored sprinkles, cheese, and Italian seasoning together in a 1-gallon zip-top bag.
- Coat both sides of the biscuits lightly with nonfat cooking spray.
- Place the biscuits in the bag and shake gently until coated with the mixture.
- Arrange the biscuits onto the prepared baking sheet.
- Sprinkle the remaining crumb mixture on top of the biscuits.
- Bake on the top rack of the oven for 8 minutes or until golden brown.

Yield: 10 (1-biscuit) servings

Calories: 64 (19% fat); Total Fat: 1 gm; Cholesterol: 2 mg; Carbohydrate: 11 gm;
Dietary Fiber: 0 gm; Protein: 2 gm; Sodium: 298 mg
Diabetic Exchanges: ½ starch

Preparation time: 7 minutes or less
Cooking time: 8 minutes or less
Total time: 15 minutes or less

Menu Idea: These are superb with any light dinner. I like serving Chicken à la King (page 121) from *Busy People's Slow Cooker Cookbook* over these instead of having just plain ol' boring biscuits.

Parmesan Garlic Biscuits

These biscuits are crunchy with a light garlic flavor.

1	(10-count) can buttermilk biscuits (I use Pillsbury)	1	teaspoon minced garlic
1	tablespoon imitation butter-flavored sprinkles	2	tablespoons finely grated Parmesan cheese

- Preheat the oven to 425 degrees. Coat a baking sheet with nonfat cooking spray.
- Arrange the biscuits over the baking sheet.
- Sprinkle the tops of the biscuits with the butter-flavored sprinkles. Spread with the garlic and lightly sprinkle each biscuit with Parmesan cheese.
- Bake for 8 minutes or until golden brown.

Yield: 10 (1-biscuit) servings

Calories: 58 (16% fat); Total Fat: 1 gm; Cholesterol: 1 mg; Carbohydrate: 10 gm; Dietary Fiber: 0 gm; Protein: 2 gm; Sodium: 239 mg
Diabetic Exchanges: $\frac{1}{2}$ starch

Preparation time: 7 minutes or less
Cooking time: 8 minutes
Total time: 15 minutes or less

Menu Idea: Have dinner waiting for you when you arrive home by serving a delicious pot of Chicken and Potato Stew (page 124) from *Busy People's Slow Cooker Cookbook* with only 199 calories per serving. Serve these biscuits with Cucumber Salad with Bacon & Blue Cheese (page 148) in this book on the side, for a great meal.

Mushroom Pinwheel Biscuits

These are extra special for extra special meals.

1 (10-ounce) can prepared pizza dough (I use Pillsbury)	³/₄ cup finely chopped fresh mushrooms
¹/₂ cup finely shredded Parmesan cheese	1 tablespoon dried parsley

- Preheat the oven to 425 degrees. Coat an 11 x 17-inch baking sheet with nonfat cooking spray.
- With your hands, spread the pizza dough to the edges of the pan.
- Sprinkle the cheese, mushrooms, and parsley over the dough.
- Starting with the long side, roll the dough and seal the edge and ends.
- Using a very sharp knife, carefully cut it into 12 slices.
- Arrange the pinwheels onto the prepared baking sheet with each biscuit laying flat on its side so you can see the pinwheel on top, making sure that the biscuits do not touch each other.
- Bake for 8 minutes or until the tops are golden brown.

Yield: 12 (1-biscuit) servings

Calories: 77 (24% fat); Total Fat: 2 gm; Cholesterol: 3 mg; Carbohydrate: 11 gm; Dietary Fiber: 0 gm; Protein: 4 gm; Sodium: 222 mg
Diabetic Exchanges: ¹/₂ starch

Preparation time: 7 minutes
Cooking time: 8 minutes
Total time: 15 minutes

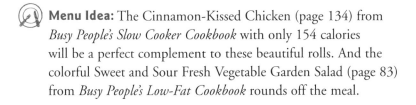

Menu Idea: The Cinnamon-Kissed Chicken (page 134) from *Busy People's Slow Cooker Cookbook* with only 154 calories will be a perfect complement to these beautiful rolls. And the colorful Sweet and Sour Fresh Vegetable Garden Salad (page 83) from *Busy People's Low-Fat Cookbook* rounds off the meal.

Candy Cane Biscuits

These cherry biscuits shaped like candy canes are festive for Christmas meals.

15	maraschino cherries, finely chopped	1	tablespoon vanilla frosting (I use Snackwell's)
1	(10-count) can buttermilk biscuits (I use Pillsbury)	2	tablespoons sugar
		2	drops red food coloring

- Preheat the oven to 425 degrees. Coat a baking sheet with nonfat cooking spray.
- Press the chopped cherries into the biscuits.
- Twist and roll each biscuit with your hands into a rope.
- Shape the ropes into canes.
- Arrange the biscuits on the prepared baking sheet and bake for 8 minutes or until the bottoms are golden brown.
- Microwave the frosting for 10 seconds or until hot and bubbly. Drizzle the frosting over the warm biscuits.
- In a small bowl, mix the sugar with the red food coloring.
- Sprinkle the sugar over the biscuits and serve warm.

Yield: 10 (1-biscuit) servings

Calories: 82 (11% fat); Total Fat: 1 gm; Cholesterol: 0 mg; Carbohydrate: 16 gm; Dietary Fiber: 0 gm; Protein: 1 gm; Sodium: 168 mg
Diabetic Exchanges: 1 starch

Preparation time: 17 minutes or less
Cooking time: 8 minutes or less
Total time: 25 minutes or less

Menu Ideas: The fun candy cane–shaped biscuits are perfect for Christmas morning with Rainbow Fresh-Fruit Salad (page 136) in this book or a breakfast bake such as the Mushroom and Onion Frittata (page 91) from *Busy People's Down-Home Cooking Without the Down-Home Fat.*

Cranberry Corn Muffins

Good for any time of the day: breakfast, snack, lunch, or dinner.

1 (8.5-ounce) package Jiffy corn muffin mix, dry (do not prepare as directed on box)	2 egg whites
1/3 cup water	1/3 cup shredded fat-free Cheddar cheese
	1/3 cup chopped dried cranberries

- Preheat the oven to 350 degrees. Coat 10 muffin cups with nonfat cooking spray.
- Combine the corn muffin mix, water, and egg whites in a bowl. The batter will be lumpy.
- Stir in the cheese and chopped cranberries.
- Fill the prepared muffin tins half full.
- Bake for 15 to 17 minutes or until golden brown.

Yield: 10 (1-muffin) servings

Calories: 133 (29% fat); Total Fat: 4 gm; Cholesterol: 4 mg; Carbohydrate: 20 gm; Dietary Fiber: 2 gm; Protein: 3 gm; Sodium: 302 mg
Diabetic Exchanges: 1 starch, $1/2$ fruit, 1 fat

Preparation time: 8 minutes
Cooking time: 17 minutes or less
Total time: 25 minutes or less

Menu Ideas: These are yummy with a turkey or pork tenderloin dinner. They are also tasty with breakfast entrées such as scrambled eggs made with liquid egg substitute.

Raisin Bran Muffins

Great to keep on hand for those "on-the-go rushed mornings" when sitting down for breakfast isn't an option.

1 ¼ cups all-purpose flour	1 cup skim milk
1 tablespoon baking powder	2 egg whites
⅓ cup packed dark brown sugar	¼ cup applesauce
1 ¼ cups raisin bran cereal	

- Preheat the oven to 400 degrees. Coat 12 muffin cups with nonfat cooking spray.
- Combine the flour, baking powder, and brown sugar in a bowl.
- In a large bowl combine the cereal and milk and let it sit for 2 minutes.
- Stir the egg whites and applesauce into the cereal until well mixed.
- Add the dry ingredients and stir until well blended.
- Spoon the batter into the prepared muffin cups.
- Bake for 20 minutes or until golden brown.

Yield: 12 (1-muffin) servings

Calories: 101 (0% fat); Total Fat: 0 gm; Cholesterol: 0 mg; Carbohydrate: 22 gm; Dietary Fiber: 1 gm; Protein: 3 gm; Sodium: 182 mg
Diabetic Exchanges: 1½ starch

Preparation time: 10 minutes or less
Cooking time: 20 minutes
Total time: 30 minutes or less

Menu Ideas: These muffins go well with the Broccoli, Ham & Cheese Frittata (page 39) and the Fake Bacon (page 30), both from *Busy People's Low-Fat Cookbook*.

Pumpkin Muffins

Delicious!

1 **(15-ounce) can solid pumpkin (not spiced pie filling)**	1 **(16-ounce) package angel food cake mix, dry (do not prepare as directed on box)**
2 **teaspoons pumpkin pie spice**	
¼ **cup water**	

- Preheat the oven to 350 degrees.
- Coat 24 regular-size muffin cups with nonfat cooking spray.
- In a large bowl combine the pumpkin, pumpkin pie spice, and water together until well mixed.
- Gradually stir in the cake mix and continue to stir until all the ingredients are well blended (batter will poof up).
- Fill the prepared muffin cups half full.
- Bake for 15 minutes or until a toothpick inserted in the center of a muffin comes out clean.

Yield: 24 (1-muffin) servings

Calories: 76 (0% fat); Total Fat: 0 gm; Cholesterol: 0 mg; Carbohydrate: 17 gm;
Dietary Fiber: 1 gm; Protein: 2 gm; Sodium: 165 mg
Diabetic Exchanges: 1 other carbohydrate

Preparation time: 10 minutes
Cooking time: 15 minutes
Total time: 25 minutes

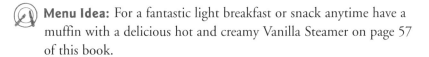

Menu Idea: For a fantastic light breakfast or snack anytime have a muffin with a delicious hot and creamy Vanilla Steamer on page 57 of this book.

Piña Colada Muffins

This is a light and airy tropical flavored muffin.

1 **(20-ounce) can crushed pineapple, undrained**	1 **(16-ounce) angel food cake mix, dry (do not make as directed on box)**
1 ½ **teaspoons coconut extract**	¼ **cup shredded coconut**

- Preheat the oven to 350 degrees.
- Coat 36 regular-size muffin cups with nonfat cooking spray.
- Reserve 1 cup of the pineapple juice. Discard the remaining juice.
- Stir the crushed pineapple, pineapple juice, and coconut extract together in a bowl until well mixed.
- Add the cake mix, stirring until the ingredients are combined.
- Spoon the batter into the prepared muffin tins, filling each ½ full.
- Sprinkle the shredded coconut over the top of the batter.
- Bake for 15 minutes or until a toothpick inserted in the center of a muffin comes out clean.

Yield: 36 (1-muffin) servings

Calories: 56 (4% fat); Total Fat: trace; Cholesterol: 0 mg; Carbohydrate: 2 gm; Dietary Fiber: 0 gm; Protein: 1 gm; Sodium: 112 mg
Diabetic Exchanges: 1 other carbohydrate

Preparation time: 10 minutes
Cooking time: 15 minutes
Total time: 25 minutes

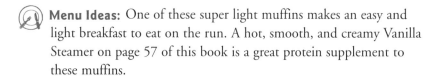

Menu Ideas: One of these super light muffins makes an easy and light breakfast to eat on the run. A hot, smooth, and creamy Vanilla Steamer on page 57 of this book is a great protein supplement to these muffins.

Apple Muffins

This easy recipe is nice because it saves us time by not having to peel the apples ourselves. If it can save me time, I like that!

1	(20-ounce) can Comstock sliced apples (not pie filling), undrained	1	(16-ounce) angel food cake mix, dry (do not make as directed on box)
¼	cup water	2	tablespoons Splenda Granular
1	teaspoon plus 1 teaspoon ground cinnamon		

- Preheat the oven to 350 degrees.
- Coat 24 regular-size muffin cups with nonfat cooking spray.
- Using a long knife, cut the apples into small pieces while they are still in the can. (This saves time and also saves having to clean another dish.)
- In a medium bowl, mix the apples, water, and 1 teaspoon of the cinnamon until well blended.
- Stir in the cake mix until well mixed.
- Fill the prepared muffin tins half full.
- Mix the Splenda with the remaining 1 teaspoon cinnamon. Sprinkle the mixture lightly over the tops of the muffins before baking.
- Bake for 20 minutes or until a toothpick inserted in the center of a muffin comes out clean.

Yield: 24 (1-muffin) servings

Calories: 80 (0% fat); Total Fat: 0 gm; Cholesterol: 0 mg; Carbohydrate: 18 gm; Dietary Fiber: 1 gm; Protein: 2 gm; Sodium: 167 mg
Diabetic Exchanges: 1 other carbohydrate

Preparation time: 5 minutes
Cooking time: 20 minutes
Total time: 25 minutes

Menu Idea: The Café Latte recipe on page 58 of this book goes great with these muffins and is also a good source of hidden protein for your morning start or afternoon "pick-me-up" snack.

Buttermilk Cornbread Muffins

These muffins are just right for people who do not like sweet cornbread. These are not sweet at all.

3 tablespoons unsweetened applesauce	2 tablespoons Splenda Granular
1 1/2 cups low-fat buttermilk	2 cups self-rising cornmeal mix
1/4 cup liquid egg substitute or 2 egg whites	

- Preheat the oven to 425 degrees.
- Coat 12 medium-size muffin cups with nonfat cooking spray.
- In a medium mixing bowl using a spatula, mix together the applesauce, buttermilk, egg substitute, and Splenda until well blended.
- Stir in the cornmeal. Continue stirring until well mixed.
- Pour 1/3 cup batter into each prepared muffin cup.
- Bake for 15 minutes or until a knife inserted in the center comes out clean.

Yield: 12 (1-muffin) servings

Calories: 115 (9% fat); Total Fat: 1 gm; Cholesterol: 1 mg; Carbohydrate: 23 gm; Dietary Fiber: 2 gm; Protein: 3 gm; Sodium: 452 mg
Diabetic Exchanges: 1 1/2 starch

Preparation time: 5 minutes
Cooking time: 15 minutes or less
Total time: 20 minutes or less

Menu Idea: The Southwestern Vegetarian Soup on page 59 of *Busy People's Slow Cooker Cookbook* complements the taste and texture of these muffins.

Black & Blue Berry Muffins

The fun recipe name came by combining blackberries with blueberries for a delicious blend of berries, which is exceptionally good when berries are in season.

1/3 cup applesauce
1/4 cup liquid egg substitute
1/4 cup skim milk
1 1/2 cups reduced-fat baking mix
 (I use Bisquick)

3/4 cup plus I tablespoon Splenda
1/2 cup fresh blueberries
1/2 cup fresh blackberries

- Preheat the oven to 400 degrees.
- In a medium bowl, stir together the applesauce, egg substitute, and skim milk until well mixed.
- Stir in the baking mix and ¾ cup of the Splenda, mixing well.
- Gently fold in the blueberries and blackberries. Mix just enough to get them evenly scattered throughout the batter.
- Line 12 regular-size muffin cups with cupcake liners and coat the liners with nonfat cooking spray. Fill each cup three-quarters full with batter.
- Bake for 18 to 20 minutes or until a toothpick inserted in the center of a muffin comes out clean.
- Let cool a few minutes. Coat the top of the muffins with nonfat cooking spray and lightly sprinkle with the remaining 1 tablespoon Splenda.
- If desired, you can also sprinkle the tops of the muffins lightly with ground cinnamon or cinnamon sugar.

Yield: 12 (1-muffin) servings

Calories: 77 (12% fat); Total Fat: 1 gm; Cholesterol: 0 mg; Carbohydrate: 15 gm; Dietary Fiber: 1 gm; Protein: 2 gm; Sodium: 188 mg
Diabetic Exchanges: 1 starch

Preparation time: 5 minutes
Cooking time: 20 minutes or less
Total time: 25 minutes or less

Menu Idea: For a quickie breakfast on the run, these taste great with Very Cherry Protein Drink on page 43 of this book.

Breakfast Pizza

This is a great way to start the day.

1 **(10-ounce) can prepared pizza crust (I use Pillsbury)**	1/2 **cup liquid egg substitute**
1 **cup finely chopped fully-cooked lean ham**	1 **(12-ounce) container fat-free sour cream**
2 **cups shredded fat-free Swiss or mozzarella cheese (I use Kraft)**	1/2 **cup chopped fresh or frozen onion**

- Preheat the oven to 425 degrees. Coat an 11 x 17-inch jelly roll pan with nonfat cooking spray.
- With your hands, spread the pizza crust to the edges of the pan. Arrange the ham and cheese over the crust.
- In a medium bowl beat the egg substitute, sour cream, and onion together with a spoon until well blended. Pour over the ham and cheese.
- Bake for 17 to 20 minutes or until the pizza crust is golden brown. Cut into squares and serve.

Yield: 8 servings

Calories: 198 (12% fat); Total Fat: 3 gm; Cholesterol: 15 mg; Carbohydrate: 24 gm; Dietary Fiber: 1 gm; Protein: 18 gm; Sodium: 741 mg
Diabetic Exchanges: 2 very lean meat, 1 1/2 starch

Preparation time: 10 minutes
Cooking time: 20 minutes or less
Total time: 30 minutes or less

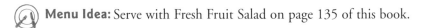 **Menu Idea:** Serve with Fresh Fruit Salad on page 135 of this book.

Lemon Breakfast Bake

This is so yummy, you may not want to serve it just for breakfast. It's also good for after-school snacks.

1 (7.5-ounce) can buttermilk biscuits (I use Pillsbury)	1/2 cup sugar
1 (8-ounce) package fat-free cream cheese, softened	2 egg whites
	1/2 teaspoon lemon extract

- Preheat the oven to 375 degrees. Coat a 9 x 13-inch baking dish with nonfat cooking spray.
- With your hands, flatten the biscuits into the bottom of the prepared baking dish, forming them together to cover the entire dish.
- With a mixer, beat the cream cheese, sugar, egg whites, and lemon extract together until well mixed.
- Spoon the filling over the top of the biscuit layer and bake for 20 minutes.

Yield: 20 servings

Calories: 57 (6% fat); Total Fat: trace; Cholesterol: 1 mg; Carbohydrate: 11 gm; Dietary Fiber: 0 gm; Protein: 3 gm; Sodium: 143 mg
Diabetic Exchanges: 1/2 other carbohydrate

Preparation time: 5 minutes
Cooking time: 20 minutes
Total time: 25 minutes

Menu Idea: I love the Vanilla Steamer (page 57) in this book with these treats.

Breakfast Parfait

This is one of my all-time favorites. It's good any time of the day.

I (8-ounce) container sugar-free, fat-free yogurt—any flavor (I like strawberry)

I small banana, cut into thin slices

$1/2$ cup 98% fat-free granola (I use Health Valley)

- Spoon half the yogurt into the bottom of two pretty parfait glasses. (If you don't have parfait glasses, any widemouthed 10-ounce glass will be fine.)
- Top with half the banana slices.
- Sprinkle half the granola over the banana slices.
- Repeat the layers with the remaining yogurt, banana slices, and granola.
- If you like, reserve a small amount of yogurt to top off each dessert.

Yield: 2 ($1\frac{1}{4}$-cup) servings

Calories: 135 (0% fat); Total Fat: 0 gm; Cholesterol: 2 mg; Carbohydrate: 28 gm; Dietary Fiber: 3 gm; Protein: 7 gm; Sodium: 100 mg
Diabetic Exchanges: 1 starch, 1 skim milk

Preparation time: 5 minutes

Menu Idea: A meal in itself. However, for added nutrition have a Raisin Bran Muffin (page 80) in this book.

Breakfast Trifle

Vonda and Todd (D.J.s for YES FM, 89.3 in Toledo, Ohio) gave this "Two big thumbs up!"

1	**(32-ounce) container sugar free, fat-free strawberry yogurt**	**1 pound fresh strawberries, halved**
1	**(12 ½-ounce) box 98% fat-free granola (I use Health Valley)**	**1 (32-ounce) container sugar-free, fat-free vanilla yogurt**

- Spread the strawberry yogurt in the bottom of a glass bowl.
- Sprinkle half the granola over the yogurt.
- Arrange the strawberries on top.
- Spread the vanilla yogurt over the strawberries.
- Sprinkle the remaining granola on top. Serve chilled.

Note: Bananas, blueberries, or any other kind of fruit can be substituted to make an array of different Breakfast Trifle combinations.

Yield: 15 (6-ounce) servings

Calories: 148 (4% fat); Total Fat: 1 gm; Cholesterol: 2 mg; Carbohydrate: 30 gm; Dietary Fiber: 4 gm; Protein: 8 gm; Sodium: 109 mg
Diabetic Exchanges: 1 starch, 1 skim milk

Preparation time: 5 minutes or less

Menu Ideas: This is super served on breakfast or brunch buffets.

Buttermilk Pancake Squares

These remind me of mini buttermilk pancakes but without all the fuss and time. They're very good with just a little reduced-calorie maple syrup, or you can just eat them warm from the oven as is. If you are serving a big crowd for brunch or breakfast and don't want to stand behind a hot stove for a long time flipping a bunch of small pancakes, here's your answer.

2 cups low-fat buttermilk	1 tablespoon imitation butter-flavor sprinkles (I use Molly McButter)
3/4 cup Splenda Granular	
1 1/2 cups reduced-fat baking mix (I use Bisquick)	1 cup liquid egg substitute or 8 egg whites
	2 teaspoons vanilla extract

- Preheat the oven to 350 degrees.
- Coat an 11 x 17-inch jelly roll pan with nonfat cooking spray.
- In a large mixing bowl beat the buttermilk, Splenda, baking mix, butter-flavor sprinkles, egg substitute, and vanilla together until well blended.
- Pour into the prepared pan.
- Bake for 15 minutes or until a knife inserted into the center comes out clean.
- Let cool a few minutes and cut with a very sharp knife into 24 squares. Serve warm.

Yield: 8 (3-square) servings

Calories: 139 (13% fat); Total Fat: 2 gm; Cholesterol: 2 mg; Carbohydrate: 23 gm; Dietary Fiber: 0 gm; Protein: 7 gm; Sodium: 433 mg
Diabetic Exchanges: 1 1/2 starch

Preparation time: 10 minutes or less
Cooking time: 15 minutes
Total time: 25 minutes or less

Menu Idea: For a special breakfast or brunch everyone will remember, serve with extra lean grilled ham steaks, scrambled eggs made with egg substitute and topped with fresh parsley, and a fresh fruit salad of assorted berries and melons sprinkled with Splenda.

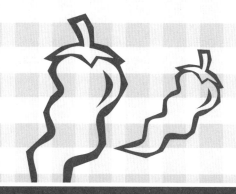

Awesome Appetizers

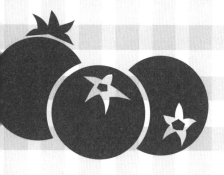

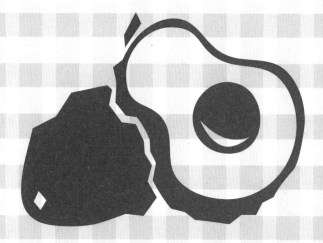

Bacon & Onion Cheese Ball

I took this to a New Year's Eve party and nobody could believe it was low fat or low calorie!

¹/₂ cup reduced-fat real bacon bits	¹/₄ cup blue cheese crumbles
¹/₂ cup fat-free sour cream	¹/₂ cup chopped green onions
1 (8-ounce) package fat-free cream cheese, softened	

- Combine the bacon bits, sour cream, cream cheese, blue cheese, and green onions in a large bowl. Stir together until well mixed.
- Shape into a ball, wrap in plastic, and chill for 1 hour before serving.

Yield: 20 (2-tablespoon) servings

Calories: 38 (30% fat); Total Fat: 1 gm; Cholesterol: 6 mg; Carbohydrate: 2 gm;
Dietary Fiber: 0 gm; Protein: 4 gm; Sodium: 185 mg
Diabetic Exchanges: ¹/₂ lean meat

Preparation time: 15 minutes

Menu Ideas: This is a good spread on celery or fat-free crackers. This complements the Cool & Creamy Spicy Tortilla Dip (page 17), Vegetable Pizza (page 27), and Spinach Balls (page 21) all from *Busy People's Down-Home Cooking Without the Down-Home Fat.*

Stuffed Mushroom Caps

These are so good that I ended up eating them as a meal even though they are supposed to be either a side dish or an appetizer.

1/4 cup reduced-fat real bacon bits	2 tablespoons crumbled blue cheese
1 (8-ounce) package fat-free cream cheese, softened	1 pound fresh medium mushrooms, stems removed
1/4 cup chopped green onions	

- Preheat the oven to 350 degrees.
- Coat a 9 x 13-inch casserole dish with nonfat cooking spray.
- Stir together the bacon bits, cream cheese, green onions, and blue cheese in a medium bowl until well mixed.
- Fill the inside of each mushroom cap with the cheese mixture.
- Cover with foil and bake for about 20 minutes or until the mushrooms are tender.

Yield: 8 servings (about 3 mushrooms per serving)

Calories: 69 (22% fat); Total Fat: 2 gm; Cholesterol: 9 mg; Carbohydrate: 5 gm; Dietary Fiber: 1 gm; Protein: 8 gm; Sodium: 298 mg
Diabetic Exchanges: 1 vegetable, 1 lean meat

Preparation time: 10 minutes
Cooking time: 20 minutes
Total time: 30 minutes

Menu Idea: These are good not only as an appetizer but also as a vegetable side dish with Chicken & Pasta Casserole (page 123) from *Busy People's Slow Cooker Cookbook* and a fresh garden salad.

Toasted Baguette Slices with Rosemary & Garlic

The herbs are enchanting and will make any ordinary meal a little more special.

1 **baguette***	1/2 **teaspoon garlic salt**
Nonfat butter spray (not cooking spray)	1 **teaspoon dried parsley**
1 **teaspoon dried rosemary**	2 **tablespoons finely shredded Parmesan cheese**

- Preheat the oven to 450 degrees.
- Cut the baguette vertically into 12 half-inch-wide slices.
- Coat both sides of each slice with 2 to 3 sprays of butter spray.
- Arrange the slices on a baking sheet.
- Lightly sprinkle the rosemary, garlic salt, and parsley on top of the bread slices.
- Sprinkle the cheese over the top.
- Bake on the top rack of the oven for 2 to 3 minutes or until the cheese is melted and golden brown.
- Serve immediately.

Note: A baguette is a long, thin loaf of French bread that is usually crispy on the outside with a soft and chewy interior texture. Most grocery stores and bakeries keep them in stock.

Yield: 4 (3-slice) servings

Calories: 89 (16% fat); Total Fat: 2 gm; Cholesterol: 2 mg; Carbohydrate: 15 gm; Dietary Fiber: 1 gm; Protein: 4 gm; Sodium: 336 mg
Diabetic Exchanges: 1 starch

Preparation time: 5 minutes or less
Cooking time: 3 minutes or less
Total time: 8 minutes or less

Menu Idea: These dress up the Chicken & Green Bean Casserole on page 159 of *Busy People's Low-Fat Cookbook* quite nicely.

Homemade Crêpes—Skinny Style

When you experience how easy crêpes (super-thin pancakes made with a real thin batter) are to prepare, you may never pay the high price for premade, prepackaged crêpes again.

1 cup all-purpose flour	2 tablespoons light butter, melted
1 1/4 cups skim milk	1 tablespoon Splenda granular
4 egg whites or 1/2 cup egg substitute	

- Combine the flour, milk, egg whites or egg substitute, butter, and Splenda in a bowl. Stir until thin and smooth. If the batter is too thick, add more milk, 1 tablespoon at a time.
- Preheat a nonstick 9-inch skillet over medium heat to the point where a drop of water on the skillet will dance and sizzle. Once the skillet is hot enough, spray it with nonfat cooking spray before putting the batter in for each crêpe. You can only make one crêpe at a time.
- Pour 1/4 cup batter into the skillet and swirl to cover the entire bottom. The batter will almost immediately dry as it touches the pan.
- Cook the crêpe only until the batter is dry in the center, which will take less than 1 minute. Turn the crêpe over with a spatula and cook for another 10 to 15 seconds, just enough to make it very lightly golden. You want the crêpe to be soft and thin, not crispy.
- Place the cooked crêpes, one at a time, in a stack on a plate, putting a sheet of wax paper between each crêpe to make separating them easier.

Note: You can make a bunch of crêpes beforehand and store them in a sealable bag with all of the air released in the refrigerator until ready to use. Simply microwave about 10 crêpes at a time for 10 to 15 seconds to warm before filling.

Yield: About 16 crêpes (1 crêpe per serving)

Calories: 46 (17% fat); Total Fat: 1 gm; Cholesterol: 3 mg; Carbohydrate: 7 gm; Dietary Fiber: 0 gm; Protein: 3 gm; Sodium: 33 mg
Diabetic Exchanges: $\frac{1}{2}$ starch

Preparation time: 5 minutes or less
Cooking time: 15 minutes or less
Total Time: 20 minutes or less

Menu Ideas: For a winning entrée, use this crêpe recipe for the delicious and savory Chicken & Broccoli Crêpes recipe on the following page. As a melt-in-your-mouth dessert, fill each crêpe with 2 tablespoons of the Butterscotch Cream Dessert Dip recipe on page 266 or the banana cream variation. Sprinkle powdered sugar very lightly on top to make them look pretty.

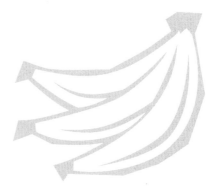

Chicken & Broccoli Crêpes

When I have an idea for a recipe, I usually have an idea of how I want it to taste. Sometimes, like this time, the recipe tastes even better than I anticipated. I am thrilled with the savory flavor of these crêpes.

1 pound frozen broccoli florets or pieces	1/2 cup fat-free mayonnaise
1 cup chopped fresh red, orange, or yellow bell pepper	1 (10 3/4-ounce) can 98% fat-free cream of celery soup
1 (13-ounce) can chicken breast in water, undrained	1/2 teaspoon dried tarragon
	1 (5-ounce) package of 10- to 9-inch crêpes*

- In a 12-inch nonstick skillet over medium-high heat cook the broccoli, covered, in 1/2 cup of water for 8 minutes.
- Add the bell pepper. Turn off the heat. Let sit, covered, for 1 to 2 minutes or until the bell pepper is tender. Drain.
- Return the skillet to the stovetop over medium heat. Move the bell pepper and broccoli to one side of the skillet.
- On the empty side of the skillet, stir together the chicken, mayonnaise, soup, and tarragon until well mixed.
- Once mixed, gently stir the pepper and broccoli into the chicken and cream mixture. Let cook, stirring frequently, for 3 to 4 minutes or until the entire dish is fully heated.
- Microwave the stack of 10 crêpes (with wax paper or divider sheets between each crêpe) for about 1 minute or until warm.
- Arrange 1 crêpe on each plate and spoon 1/3 cup of chicken and broccoli mixture down the center of each crêpe. Roll the crêpe and repeat until all the crêpes are used.
- Put either 2 crêpes on each individual plate or arrange a row of crêpes on a long serving platter. Spoon 2 tablespoons of the chicken and broccoli mixture on top of each rolled crêpe.
- Serve immediately. If the crêpes cool too much before serving, microwave each crêpe for 5 to 10 seconds to reheat.
- If a fancier presentation is desired, very lightly sprinkle the tops of the crêpes with paprika.

Note: For faster preparation you can purchase crêpes from the grocery store. However, they are more expensive than homemade. For homemade crêpes, follow the recipe on page 96.

Yield: 5 (2-crêpe) servings

Calories: 220 (20% fat); Total Fat: 5 gm; Cholesterol: 45 mg; Carbohydrate: 25 gm; Dietary Fiber: 4 gm; Protein: 18 gm; Sodium: 1008 mg
Diabetic Exchanges: 1 starch, 2 vegetable, 2 lean meat

Preparation time: 8 minutes
Cooking time: 17 minutes or less
Total Time: 25 minutes or less

Menu Idea: These make a great meal anytime—breakfast, brunch, lunch, or dinner. The Spiced Apples (page 112) from *Busy People's Slow Cooker Cookbook* complement and finish this meal beautifully.

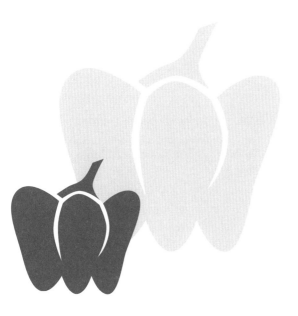

Bean Dip

My family likes this homemade bean dip every bit as much as the store-bought kind, and it's a fraction of the cost! The key is to buy the least expensive ingredients possible to make this recipe. You can't taste the difference, and you'll save mucho moola! (A lot of money!)

I (16-ounce) can fat-free refried beans	**2 teaspoons taco seasoning mix**

- Mix the refried beans and taco seasoning mix together in a bowl using a spatula until well blended. Serve at room temperature. Refrigerate any unused portion.

Yield: 10 (¼-cup) servings

Calories: 38; Total Fat: 0 gm; Percent Fat Calories: 0%; Cholesterol: 0 mg; Carbohydrate: 7 gm; Dietary Fiber: 2 gm; Protein: 2 gm; Sodium: 191 mg
Diabetic Exchanges: ½ starch

Preparation time: 5 minutes or less

Cheesy Bean Dip:
Prepare the Bean Dip, stirring in ½ cup of heated Cheez Whiz Light. Serve at room temperature.

Yield: 12 (¼-cup) servings

Calories: 56; Total Fat: 1 gm; Percent Fat Calories: 18%; Cholesterol: 4 mg; Carbohydrate: 8 gm; Dietary Fiber: 2 gm; Protein: 4 gm; Sodium: 358 mg
Diabetic Exchanges: ½ starch

Menu Ideas: Serve with Baked Tostitos or Baked Bugles. For a Mexican-themed meal, serve as an appetizer with low-calorie Mexican foods such as Taco Vegetable Soup (page 71) from *Busy People's Low-Fat Cookbook* and a bowl of assorted fresh green lettuces topped with a serving of Cool & Creamy Spicy Tortilla Dip (page 17) from *Busy People's Down-Home Cooking Without the Down-Home Fat* as a dressing.

Southwestern Refried Bean Dip

This thick dip is very rich and tasty.

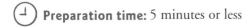

I (1.25-ounce) package taco seasoning mix	I (16-ounce) can fat-free refried beans
I (16-ounce) container fat-free sour cream	Tabasco (optional)

- In a bowl, combine the taco seasoning mix and sour cream.
- Stir in the refried beans.
- Serve as is or chilled.
- For those liking spicier foods, add a few drops of Tabasco sauce to taste.

Yield: 14 ($\frac{1}{4}$-cup) servings

Calories: 64; Total Fat: 0 gm; Percent Fat Calories: 0%; Cholesterol: 3 mg; Carbohydrate: 11 gm; Dietary Fiber: 2 gm; Protein: 3 gm; Sodium: 259 mg
Diabetic Exchanges: $\frac{1}{2}$ starch

Preparation time: 5 minutes or less

Menu Ideas: Serve with Baked Tostitos. For a Mexican-themed party serve with these other southwestern appetizers: South of the Border Cheese Spread (page 33) from *Busy People's Down-Home Cooking Without the Down-Home Fat* and Mexican Confetti Dip (page 30) and Taco Chowder (page 74) both from *Busy People's Slow Cooker Cookbook.*

Pumpkin Dip

This is a terrific way to get children to want to eat nutritious food without their even knowing it! Children love to dip their food into special treats.

1 cup cold water	1 cup canned solid pumpkin
1 (1-ounce) box sugar-free, fat-free instant butterscotch pudding mix, dry (do not make as directed on box)	1 teaspoon pumpkin pie spice
	2 to 3 individual packets Splenda

- In a medium mixing bowl beat together the water and pudding mix with an electric mixer until thick and well blended.
- Add the pumpkin, pumpkin pie spice, and Splenda. Continue mixing until well blended.
- Refrigerate until ready to use.

Yield: 12 (2-tablespoon) servings

Calories: 15 (0% fat); Total Fat: 0 gm; Cholesterol: 0 mg; Carbohydrate: 3 gm;
Dietary Fiber: 1 gm; Protein: 0 gm; Sodium: 99 mg
Diabetic Exchanges: Free

Preparation time: 5 minutes or less

Menu Idea: Serve with animal crackers, reduced-fat crackers, or reduced-fat graham crackers for dipping.

Spicy & Creamy Sausage Dip

I converted an extremely high-fat appetizer recipe (from my girlfriend Kim Hohlbein) into this fantastic, healthy version that nobody would ever guess is low fat or vegetarian. Plus, I made it in a fraction of the time it took her to make her unhealthy recipe. Does life get any better than this, folks?

1 (12-ounce) bag sausage-flavored Ground Meatless crumbles (I use Morningstar Farms)

1 (14½-ounce) can diced tomatoes with green chilies

2 (8-ounce) packages fat-free cream cheese, softened

■ Heat a 12-inch nonstick skillet over medium-low heat. Add the veggie crumbles, tomatoes, and cream cheese. Cook for about 5 minutes or until the cream cheese is melted and all the ingredients are heated through, stirring frequently.

Note: Ground Meatless is a vegetarian product that tastes like cooked, crumbled hamburger. It does not need to be cooked before adding to the recipe. See page 16 for more information.

Yield: 17 (¼-cup) servings

Calories: 65 (17% fat); Total Fat: 1 gm; Cholesterol: 5 mg; Carbohydrate: 5 gm; Dietary Fiber: 1 gm; Protein: 8 gm; Sodium: 363 mg
Diabetic Exchanges: 1 vegetable, 1 very lean meat

Preparation time: 5 minutes or less
Cooking time: 5 minutes or less
Total time: 10 minutes or less

Menu Idea: This is excellent served with baked tortilla chips and is perfect for parties. Keep it warm for buffets by serving the creamy dip from a slow cooker heated on low.

Warm Spinach & Bacon Dip

No need to order expensive and high-fat spinach dips at restaurants anymore when you can enjoy this in the comfort of your own home at a fraction of the cost, fat, and calories.

$1/2$ cup finely chopped onion
1 (3-ounce) jar reduced-fat real bacon bits
2 (8-ounce) packages fat-free cream cheese, softened
1 (7.75-ounce) can spinach, drained and chopped
$1/4$ cup liquid fat-free nondairy creamer

- In a saucepan over medium heat, cook the onion in 2 tablespoons of water until tender.
- Reduce the heat to medium-low.
- Stir in the bacon bits, cream cheese, spinach, and creamer. Continue cooking over medium-low heat until the cheese is melted and the texture is creamy, 5 to 7 minutes.

Yield: 24 (2-tablespoon) servings

Calories: 41 (22% fat); Total Fat: 1 gm; Cholesterol: 6 mg; Carbohydrate: 2 gm; Dietary Fiber: 0 gm; Protein: 4 gm; Sodium: 253 mg
Diabetic Exchanges: $1/2$ lean meat

Preparation time: 5 minutes or less
Cooking time: 10 minutes or less
Total time: 15 minutes or less

Menu Idea: Serve with baked tortilla chips. This is a great appetizer to start off egg-based meals such as Mushroom & Onion Frittata (page 91) from *Busy People's Down-Home Cooking Without the Down-Home Fat.*

Spinach & Artichoke Dip

This is healthy enough to be served as a vegetable dish with your meal or as an appetizer for parties. Any way you serve it, you'll agree it tastes good.

I	(10-ounce) bag frozen chopped spinach, thawed	I	(4-ounce) can chopped green chilies, undrained
I	(16-ounce) can artichoke hearts, drained and chopped	I	cup fat-free mayonnaise
		I	cup fat-free shredded mozzarella cheese

- In a medium saucepan, combine the spinach, artichokes, chilies, mayonnaise, and cheese. Cook over medium-low heat until the cheese is completely melted and all the ingredients are heated through, 5 to 7 minutes.
- Serve immediately.

Yield: 10 (¼-cup) servings

Calories: 47 (13% fat); Total Fat: 1 gm; Cholesterol: 5 mg; Carbohydrate: 6 gm; Dietary Fiber: 2 gm; Protein: 4 gm; Sodium: 450 mg
Diabetic Exchanges: ½ other carbohydrate, ½ very lean meat

Preparation time: 5 minutes or less
Cooking time: 7 minutes or less
Total time: 12 minutes or less

Menu Idea: This makes a good appetizer for dishes such as grilled or broiled fish; the Orange Roughy with Seasoned Crumb Topping recipe on page 182 in this book is a good choice.

Italian Dunkers

This recipe was created by my daughters, Whitney and Ashley. If you like pizza you'll love this!

4	hot dog buns (I like Aunt Millie) Italian seasoning	1	(14-ounce) jar pizza or pasta sauce, warmed
4	fat-free Cheddar cheese slices, cut in half		

- Halve the hot dog buns lengthwise. Sprinkle each bun with Italian seasoning.
- Arrange 1 slice of cheese on top of each bun. Microwave until the cheese softens, about 5 seconds.
- Dip the cheesy bread into the warmed pizza sauce and serve.

Yield: 8 servings

Calories: 88; Total Fat: 2 gm; Percent Fat Calories: 16%; Cholesterol: 0 mg; Carbohydrate: 15 gm; Dietary Fiber: 2 gm; Protein: 4 gm; Sodium: 328 mg
Diabetic Exchanges: 1 starch

Preparation time: 5 minutes or less

Menu Idea: This makes a great after-school snack or lunch. For a meal, serve with the Pizza Soup (page 57) from *Busy People's Slow Cooker Cookbook* and Tabbouleh Tossed Salad (page 61) from *Busy People's Down-Home Cooking Without the Down-Home Fat.*

Smoked Sausage Cheese Spread

This is a perfect dish for football parties.

1 (14-ounce) package fat-free smoked sausage (I use Butterball)	1/2 cup fat-free mayonnaise (Do not use Miracle Whip!)
	1/2 teaspoon garlic powder
3 (8-ounce) packages fat-free cream cheese, softened	1/2 teaspoon minced garlic
4 green onions, chopped	1 (1-ounce) package Ranch dip mix (found in salad dressing aisle)

- Grind the smoked sausage in a food processor until finely ground.
- In a large bowl, combine the ground sausage, cream cheese, green onions, mayonnaise, garlic powder, garlic, and Ranch dip mix. Stir with a spatula until well mixed.

Yield: 28 (2-tablespoon) servings

Calories: 43 (0% fat); Total Fat: 0 gm; Cholesterol: 9 mg; Carbohydrate: 5 gm;
Dietary Fiber: 0 gm; Protein: 6 gm; Sodium: 436 mg
Diabetic Exchanges: 1 very lean meat, 1/2 other carbohydrate

Preparation time: 10 minutes

Menu Ideas: Serve with fat-free crackers or stuffed in celery sticks or cherry tomatoes. For a party, serve with an assortment of low-calorie appetizers found in *Busy People's Down-Home Cooking Without the Down-Home Fat*, such as Portobello Garlic Mushrooms (page 13), Cool & Creamy Spicy Tortilla Dip (page 17), and Vegetable Pizza (page 27).

Hawaiian Chicken Spread

Tropical flavors make this chicken spread unique.

I	(8-ounce) package fat-free cream cheese, softened	3	tablespoons fresh chopped chives (or I ½ tablespoons dried)
I	(8-ounce) can crushed pineapple in its own juice, drained	2	tablespoons Kikkoman Teriyaki Baste and Glaze (found in barbecue sauce section)
I	(5-ounce) can chicken, drained		

- In a large bowl combine the cream cheese, pineapple, chicken, chives, and Teriyaki glaze together. Serve chilled.

Yield: 16 (2-tablespoon) servings

Calories: 35 (19% fat); Total Fat: 1 gm; Cholesterol: 7 mg; Carbohydrate: 3 gm; Dietary Fiber: 0 gm; Protein: 4 gm; Sodium: 164 mg
Diabetic Exchanges: ½ very lean meat

 Preparation time: 10 minutes

Hawaiian Tuna Spread:
Make exactly the same, but substitute 1 (6-ounce) can of tuna for the chicken.

Calories: 34 (9% fat); Total Fat: trace; Cholesterol: 6 mg; Carbohydrate: 3 gm; Dietary Fiber: 0 gm; Protein: 5 gm; Sodium: 160 mg
Diabetic Exchanges: ½ very lean meat

 Menu Ideas: This spread is good stuffed in celery or spread on crackers. For a tasty open-faced sandwich, spread over toasted bread. For lunch, stuff in a pita pocket or spread on a flour tortilla with leaf lettuce and serve as a wrap.

Crunchy Vegetable Spread

This spread is absolutely delicious and so versatile!

1 (8-ounce) package fat-free cream cheese, softened	1 cup chopped celery
	1 medium red bell pepper, chopped
1 (8-ounce) container fat-free sour cream	1 medium cucumber, seeded and chopped
1 (0.59-ounce) package Ranch dip mix, dry (I use Hidden Valley)	1/4 cup fresh or frozen chopped onion

- In a mixing bowl using an electric mixer, beat together the cream cheese, sour cream, and Ranch dip mix until well blended and creamy.
- Using a spoon, stir in the celery, bell pepper, cucumber, and onion until well blended.

Yield: 10 (¼-cup) servings

Calories: 56 (0% fat); Total Fat: 0 gm; Cholesterol: 4 mg; Carbohydrate: 8 gm; Dietary Fiber: 1 gm; Protein: 5 gm; Sodium: 332 mg
Diabetic Exchanges: 1½ vegetable

Preparation time: 10 minutes

Menu Ideas: This vegetable spread is absolutely delicious on Garlic Crisps (page 29) from *Busy People's Down-Home Cooking Without the Down-Home Fat* or on pita bread. For a complete meal serve on Garlic Crisps with Spicy Thick Vegetarian Chili (page 75) from *Busy People's Low-Fat Cookbook*.

Mushroom & Onion Cheese Spread

This creamy spread with chunks of mushrooms has a mild flavor that mushroom lovers will really like.

8 ounces fresh mushrooms, very finely diced	1 teaspoon minced garlic
$1/4$ cup chopped green onions	$1/4$ cup fat-free sour cream
1 (8-ounce) package fat-free cream cheese, softened	

- In a bowl, stir the mushrooms, green onions, cream cheese, garlic, and sour cream together until well mixed.
- Keep chilled until ready to eat.

Yield: 16 (2-tablespoon) servings

Calories: 24 (0% fat); Total Fat: 0 gm; Cholesterol: 3 mg; Carbohydrate: 3 gm; Dietary Fiber: 0 gm; Protein: 3 gm; Sodium: 74 mg
Diabetic Exchanges: $1/2$ very lean meat

Preparation time: 10 minutes

Menu Ideas: Serve on toasted bagels, bagel chips, fat-free crackers, or baked tortilla chips. Since this has a mild flavor, serve as an appetizer before an entrée that has a distinctive flavor such as Pork Chili (page 40) from *Busy People's Down-Home Cooking Without the Down-Home Fat.*

Shrimp Spread

This appetizer should be served at extra-special occasions. It is more special than just shrimp over cocktail sauce and cream cheese. It is as pretty as it is yummy!

1 plus ¹/₂ cup shredded fat-free mozzarella cheese (I use Kraft)	¹/₂ cup plus 1 tablespoon chopped fresh chives
1 (8-ounce) package fat-free cream cheese, softened	1 (8-ounce) jar cocktail sauce
1 (8-ounce) container fat-free sour cream	1 pound cooked cocktail shrimp (40/50 count), tails removed
	¹/₂ cup finely chopped tomato

- In a mixing bowl combine 1 cup of the mozzarella cheese with the cream cheese, sour cream, and ¹/₂ cup of the fresh chives. Stir until smooth.
- Spread the cheese mixture onto a cake plate.
- Cover with the cocktail sauce.
- Top with the remaining ¹/₂ cup mozzarella cheese, shrimp, the remaining 1 tablespoon chives, and tomatoes.

Note: For a seafood spread use 8 ounces cooked crab and 8 ounces cooked shrimp instead of 1 pound shrimp.

Yield: 24 (¹/₄-cup) servings

(with shrimp) Calories: 58 (7% fat); Total Fat: trace; Cholesterol: 39 mg; Carbohydrate: 5 gm; Dietary Fiber: 0 gm; Protein: 8 gm; Sodium: 280 mg Diabetic Exchanges: 1 very lean meat, ¹/₂ other carbohydrate
(with shrimp and crab) Calories: 62 (14% fat); Total Fat: 1 gm; Cholesterol: 30 mg; Carbohydrate: 5 gm; Dietary Fiber: 0 gm; Protein: 8 gm; Sodium: 289 mg Diabetic Exchanges: 1 very lean meat, ¹/₂ other carbohydrate

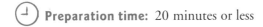 **Preparation time:** 20 minutes or less

Menu Ideas: Serve with crackers. This is a fancy way to begin an extra special meal such as Sautéed Scallops with Garlic (180) and Tangy Tossed Salad (page 95) from *Busy People's Low-Fat Cookbook* and Broccoli with Blue Cheese (page 72) from *Busy People's Down-Home Cooking Without the Down-Home Fat.*

Kickin' Chicken Spread

My secret ingredient gives this chicken spread a great little kick your guests are sure to enjoy. The secret ingredient, peanut sauce, is easy to find at your local supermarket in either the sauce or spice sections. Peanut sauce is usually used in Thai cooking.

2 tablespoons peanut sauce	I (13-ounce) can 98% fat-free chicken breast in water, drained
3 tablespoons fat-free mayonnaise dressing	2 tablespoons finely chopped red onion
I tablespoon sweet pickle relish	

- In a medium bowl stir together the peanut sauce, mayonnaise, pickle relish, chicken, and onion until well mixed.
- Keep chilled until ready to serve.

Yield: 5 (⅓-cup) servings

Calories: 108 (26% fat); Total Fat: 3 gm; Cholesterol: 31 mg; Carbohydrate: 3 gm; Dietary Fiber: 0 gm; Protein: 15 gm; Sodium: 402 mg
Diabetic Exchanges: 2 lean meat

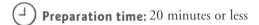 **Preparation time:** 20 minutes or less

Menu Ideas: Serve with crackers or, for a delicious and nutritious low-calorie lettuce wrap sandwich, spoon into the center of a large piece of leafy green lettuce such as romaine, iceberg, or green leaf and wrap up like a soft tortilla.

Salmon Salad Spread

The tuna really captures the flavor of the salmon in this recipe. And that's good because although it's the good fat—Omega-3 fat—salmon is high in fat. Here's a surefire winning recipe for all you salmon lovers!

2 (6-ounce) cans skinless, boneless salmon, drained	$1/2$ cup fat-free sour cream
1 (6-ounce) can tuna in water, drained	2 tablespoons Ranch salad dressing mix, dry

- Mix the salmon, tuna, sour cream, and Ranch dressing mix together in a bowl.
- Serve immediately or cover and keep refrigerated until ready to eat.

Yield: 8 ($1/4$-cup) servings

Calories: 104 (19% fat); Total Fat: 2 gm; Cholesterol: 42 mg; Carbohydrate: 4 gm; Dietary Fiber: 0 gm; Protein: 17 gm; Sodium: 535 mg
Diabetic Exchanges: $2^{1}/2$ very lean meat

Preparation time: 5 minutes or less

Menu Ideas: This is a good spread for low-fat crackers or light rye toast. I also like it on light rye Original Crispbread by Wasa. (Crispbread is like a large, crispy, dry cracker and only has 25 calories per slice.)

Ranch Stacks

This is a versatile appetizer that is satisfying enough to substitute in place of a sandwich for packed lunches.

1 **(8-ounce) package fat-free cream cheese, softened**	1/2 **cup finely chopped celery**
1 **cup fat-free sour cream**	1/4 **cup finely chopped green onions**
1 **(1-ounce) package Ranch dip mix**	9 **fat-free flour tortillas**

- With an electric mixer on medium speed, beat the cream cheese, sour cream, and Ranch dip mix together until well mixed.
- With a spoon, stir in the celery and green onions.
- Divide the mixture among six individual flour tortillas.
- Place three of the tortillas on top of the other three tortillas, clean side down, to make three stacks.
- Top each stack with a remaining tortilla.
- Press the stacks down firmly with your hands to secure together and slice each stack into six wedges.

Yield: 18 (1-wedge) servings

Calories: 72 (0% fat); Total Fat: 0 gm; Cholesterol: 2 mg; Carbohydrate: 13 gm; Dietary Fiber: 1 gm; Protein: 4 gm; Sodium: 389 mg
Diabetic Exchanges: 1 starch

Preparation time: 20 minutes or less

Menu Ideas: These make delightful appetizers or lunches. I like them as a light sandwich with a cup of soup such as my hearty Chicken Noodle Soup (page 50) from *Busy People's Slow Cooker Cookbook*.

Bagel Chips

This wonderful and easy snack was sent in by Carolyn Henderson of Howell, Michigan. Wait until you try it. You will want to make more than one.

I	onion or garlic bagel	I	teaspoon Italian seasoning
	Nonfat butter-flavored spray	1/4	teaspoon garlic salt

- Preheat the oven to 350 degrees. Coat a baking sheet with nonfat cooking spray.
- Using a serrated knife, slice the bagel vertically into thin slices.
- Arrange the slices on the baking sheet and lightly coat with butter-flavored cooking spray.
- Sprinkle the Italian seasoning and garlic salt on top.
- Bake for 12 minutes or until crispy.

Yield: 2 (½-bagel) servings

Calories: 154 (5% fat); Total Fat: 1 gm; Cholesterol: 0 mg; Carbohydrate: 30 gm;
Dietary Fiber: 1 gm; Protein: 6 gm; Sodium: 521 mg
Diabetic Exchanges: 2 starch

Preparation time: 5 minutes or less
Cooking time: 12 minutes
Total time: 17 minutes or less

Menu Ideas: These go well with Greek Pasta Salad on page 147 in this book or any fresh, tossed garden salad. I like them instead of crackers with clear broth-based soups, such as Chicken Lemon Soup on page 122 in this book.

Cheese-Filled Soft Bread Sticks

This recipe turns ordinary biscuits into extraordinary baked goods.

2 slices fat-free sharp Cheddar cheese singles (I use Kraft)	**¹/₄** cup grated Parmesan cheese
1 (7.5-ounce) can buttermilk biscuits (I use Pillsbury)	Garlic salt (optional)

- Preheat the oven to 425 degrees.
- Coat a baking sheet with nonfat cooking spray.
- Slice each cheese slice into 5 strips and make each bread stick individually as follows:
- Roll each biscuit into a rectangle roughly 4 x 1 inches.
- Lay one cheese strip down the center of each biscuit.
- Wrap each biscuit around the cheese strip. Pinch the dough at the seam to seal.
- Press the top of the bread stick into the Parmesan cheese.
- Place the bread sticks onto the baking sheet, Parmesan cheese side up. If desired, sprinkle lightly with garlic salt.
- Bake for 7 minutes or until the tops are light golden brown.

Yield: 10 bread sticks

Calories: 67 (19% fat); Total Fat: 1 gm; Cholesterol: 3 mg; Carbohydrate: 10 gm; Dietary Fiber: 0 gm; Protein: 3 gm; Sodium: 284 mg
Diabetic Exchanges: ¹/₂ starch

Preparation time: 8 minute or less
Cooking time: 7 minutes or less
Total time: 15 minutes or less

Menu Idea: Serve with any Italian meal such as Broccoli Parmesan (page 124) from *Busy People's Low-Fat Cookbook* and Rigatoni (page 184) from *Busy People's Slow Cooker Cookbook*.

Chili Cheese Cups

These south-of-the-border snacks will have you saying, "Olé!"

2 **(7.5-ounce) cans low-fat biscuits, 20 biscuits total**	¹/₂ **cup finely shredded fat-free Cheddar cheese**
I **(15-ounce) can vegetarian or turkey chili (I use Hormel)**	

- Preheat the oven to 400 degrees.
- Coat 2 baking sheets with nonfat cooking spray. Arrange the biscuits on the baking sheets and bake for 10 to 12 minutes or until golden brown.
- Cook the chili in a carousel microwave for 2 minutes or until fully heated. (If you do not have a carousel microwave, turn the dish twice during cooking.)
- Once the biscuits are baked, remove and discard the center from the biscuits. (You are making the biscuits into little cups.)
- Spoon the cooked chili into the center and return the biscuits to the baking sheets.
- Lightly sprinkle the cheese over the tops of the biscuit cups.
- Return to the oven and bake for another 2 minutes or until the cheese is melted. Serve immediately.

Yield: 20 (1-Chili Cheese Cup) servings

Calories: 77 (14% fat); Total Fat: 1 gm; Cholesterol: 4 mg; Carbohydrate: 13 gm; Dietary Fiber: 1 gm; Protein: 4 gm; Sodium: 389 mg
Diabetic Exchanges: 1 starch

Preparation time: 10 minutes or less
Cooking time: 16 minutes or less
Total time: 26 minutes or less

Menu Ideas: I like serving these either with a soup-based meal such as Southwestern Vegetable Soup (page 72) from *Busy People's Low-Fat Cookbook* or at parties as an appetizer with an assortment of other appetizers.

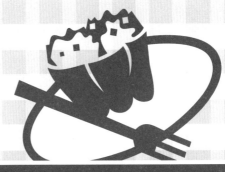

Super Easy Soups & Salads

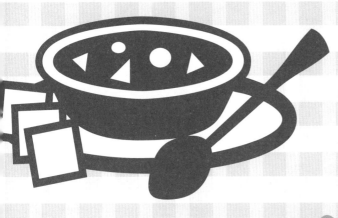

Minestrone Soup

This soup is just the way we like it: hearty and healthy.

1 **(46-ounce) can tomato juice**	1 **(15-ounce) can red kidney beans, undrained**
1 **pound eye of round, cut into tiny pieces**	2 **(14.5-ounce) cans no-salt-added stewed tomatoes, undrained**
1 **(14-ounce) jar pizza sauce (I use Ragú Family Style)**	2 **cups dry elbow macaroni**
3 **(15.25-ounce) cans mixed vegetables, undrained**	

- In a large nonstick soup pot, combine the tomato juice, eye of round, pizza sauce, mixed vegetables, beans, and tomatoes. Bring to a full boil over high heat.
- Stir in the elbow macaroni. Return to a boil. Cook, uncovered, stirring frequently for 8 minutes.

Yield: 18 (1-cup) servings

Calories: 157 (10% fat); Total Fat: 2 gm; Cholesterol: 14 mg; Carbohydrate: 25 gm; Dietary Fiber: 6 gm; Protein: 11 gm; Sodium: 617 mg
Diabetic Exchanges: 1 very lean meat, 1 starch, 2 vegetables

Preparation time: 10 minutes or less
Cooking time: 20 minutes or less
Total time: 30 minutes or less

Menu Idea: *Busy People's Down-Home Cooking Without the Down-Home Fat* has a fabulous Italian Biscuit recipe on page 28 that is so easy to whip up for this soup.

Chicken Lemon Soup

This is a perfect substitution for traditional chicken noodle soup, especially if you're feeling under the weather. As grandma would say, "It's good for what ails you."

16 cups fat-free, reduced-sodium chicken broth	1 medium onion, chopped (or 1 cup frozen chopped onion)
2 cups sliced fresh or frozen carrots (about 4 large carrots)	1 tablespoon dried parsley (or 2 tablespoons chopped fresh parsley)
1 1/2 cups chopped celery	
1 pound skinless, boneless chicken breasts, cut into bite-size pieces	1 (12-ounce) package lemon-pepper flavored penne rigate pasta (I use Pasta LaBella)

- In a large soup pot combine the chicken broth, carrots, celery, chicken, onion, and parsley. Cook over high heat, stirring occasionally.
- Once the soup has come to a roiling boil, add the pasta. Boil for 7 to 8 minutes, stirring frequently.

Yield: 20 (1-cup) servings

Calories: 114 (5% fat); Total Fat: 1 gm; Cholesterol: 13 mg; Carbohydrate: 16 gm; Dietary Fiber: 1 gm; Protein: 10 gm; Sodium: 389 mg
Diabetic Exchanges: 1 very lean meat, 1 starch

Preparation time: 10 minutes or less
Cooking time: 20 minutes or less
Total time: 30 minutes or less

Menu Idea: The Spinach Balls (page 21) from *Busy People's Down-Home Cooking Without the Down-Home Fat* are usually eaten as an appetizer, but I think they are a perfect little side dish for this soup.

Cream of Chicken & Broccoli Soup

Cream-based soups used to be off-limits for many because of their high fat content, but not anymore. Now everyone can enjoy rich, thick, and creamy soups like this one completely guilt free!

1 (10 3/4-ounce) can 98% fat-free cream of celery soup	2 cups cooked broccoli *
1 tablespoon cornstarch	1/4 cup frozen chopped onion
1 (13-ounce) can chicken breast in water, undrained	1/2 cup shredded fat-free Cheddar cheese
	5 tablespoons fat-free sour cream

- Pour the soup into a medium nonstick saucepan. Add one can full of water and the cornstarch.
- Stir together until the cornstarch is completely dissolved.
- Place the saucepan over medium heat. Add the chicken, broccoli, onion, and cheese, stirring frequently to melt the cheese and to prevent the soup from burning.
- Bring the soup to a low boil and then turn off the heat. Serve immediately by placing 1 cup of soup into each serving bowl.
- Top each serving with 1 tablespoon of the sour cream.

Note: If you do not have leftover cooked broccoli pieces, simply microwave 2 cups of broccoli pieces while preparing the soup. Stir the broccoli into the soup once the broccoli is fully cooked.

Yield: 5 (1-cup) servings

Calories: 170 (16% fat); Total Fat: 3 gm; Cholesterol: 38 mg; Carbohydrate: 13 gm; Dietary Fiber: 2 gm; Protein: 21 gm; Sodium: 815 mg
Diabetic Exchanges: 1 starch, 2 1/2 very lean meat

Preparation time: 5 minutes or less
Cooking time: 5 minutes or less
Total time: 10 minutes or less

Menu Idea: This thick and creamy soup is satisfying and filling. A small tossed salad with fat-free salad dressing, such as the Buttermilk Ranch Dressing (page 53) from *Busy People's Low-Fat Cookbook* will round off this soup into a healthy meal perfect for lunch or a light dinner.

Deluxe Bean Soup

This savory, thick, hearty soup is a winner.

2	(48-ounce) jars Randall's deluxe navy beans	2	(14-ounce) packages fat-free smoked sausage, cut into 1/4-inch pieces (I use Butterball)
8	cups fat-free no-salt-added beef broth (or 8 cups broth made from 8 bouillon cubes)	I	(10 3/4-ounce) can condensed tomato soup
I	cup frozen chopped onion	I	teaspoon dried dill weed

- Combine the beans, beef broth, and onion in a large soup pot.
- Remove 4 cups of beans and broth at a time and purée in a blender until a total of 12 cups has been puréed. Return the purée to the soup pot.
- Turn the heat on high. Add the smoked sausage, tomato soup, and dill weed. Once it is boiling, about 10 minutes, it is ready. Serve hot.

Yield: 21 (1-cup) servings

Calories: 173 (3% fat); Total Fat: 1 gm; Cholesterol: 16 mg; Carbohydrate: 27 gm; Dietary Fiber: 11 gm; Protein: 15 gm; Sodium: 1016 mg
Diabetic Exchanges: 1½ very lean meat, 2 starch

Preparation time: 10 minutes
Cooking time: 10 minutes
Total time: 20 minutes

Menu Idea: *Busy People's Down-Home Cooking Without the Down-Home Fat* has a terrific Orange Cranberry Jell-O Salad on page 46 that'd be great as a dessert after this soup for a satisfying meal.

Southwestern Stew

Here's a quick and easy south-of-the-border meatless meal you are sure to like if you like spicy foods.

1 (12-ounce) bag Ground Meatless crumbles* (I use Morningstar Farms)	1 (8-ounce) can tomato sauce
1 tablespoon dehydrated onion	1 (15-ounce) can black beans, undrained
1 (16-ounce) can creamed corn	1/2 cup salsa
	1/2 teaspoon chili powder

- In a medium saucepan over medium-high heat, stir together the Ground Meatless, onion, creamed corn, tomato sauce, black beans, salsa, and chili powder and bring to a boil.
- Lower the heat and simmer for 15 minutes or until heated through.

Note: Ground Meatless is a vegetarian product that tastes like cooked, crumbled hamburger. See page 16 for more information.

Yield: 6 (1-cup) servings

Calories: 186 (3% fat); Total Fat: 1 gm; Cholesterol: 0 mg; Carbohydrate: 32 gm; Dietary Fiber: 7 gm; Protein: 17 gm; Sodium: 1005 mg
Diabetic Exchanges: 2 starch, 2 very lean meat

Preparation time: 5 minutes
Cooking time: 15 minutes
Total time: 20 minutes

Menu Ideas: Some people like to eat this dish just as it is. It is also good served over cooked rice or polenta or with a fresh vegetable tray along with Cool & Creamy Spicy Tortilla Dip (page 17) from *Busy People's Down-Home Cooking Without the Down-Home Fat.*

Steak, Tomato & Green Chile Soup

The festive, bold flavors of this soup will complement any boring side salad or simple sandwich.

1 **(28-ounce) can low-sodium whole peeled tomatoes, undrained**	1/2 **teaspoon Mrs. Dash salt-free seasoning blend**
1 **(48-ounce) can fat-free low-sodium beef broth**	1 **pound fat-free frozen shredded hash browns**
1/2 **cup fresh or canned diced green chilies**	1/2 **pound leftover steak (grilled eye of round), cut into bite-size pieces**
	3 **individual packets Splenda**

- Cut the tomatoes into bite-size pieces while in the can.
- Combine the chopped tomatoes with juice, broth, chilies, Mrs. Dash, hash browns, and steak into a large soup pot and bring to a boil over medium-high heat.
- Boil for 5 to 10 minutes or just until the hash browns are cooked through.
- Turn off the heat. Stir in the Splenda.
- Serve hot.

Yield: 11 (1-cup) servings

Calories: 91 (9% fat); Total Fat: 1 gm; Cholesterol: 14 mg; Carbohydrate: 10 gm; Dietary Fiber: 2 gm; Protein: 11 gm; Sodium: 154 mg
Diabetic Exchanges: 1/2 starch, 1 very lean meat

Preparation time: 5 minutes
Cooking time: 15 minutes or less
Total time: 20 minutes or less

Menu Idea: Serve this with half of a lean turkey sandwich and my wonderful Dijon Mayo Spread for Sandwiches (page 56) from *Busy People's Low-Fat Cookbook.*

Seafood Bisque

My family really likes the flavor of the broth in this rich seafood treat!

2 (29-ounce) cans stew vegetables, undrained	1 pound frozen cooked shrimp, shells and tails removed
2 (10 $^3/_4$-ounce) cans 98% fat-free cream of celery soup	1 pound imitation crabmeat, cut into bite-size pieces
1 pint fat-free half-and-half	$^1/_2$ pound imitation scallops
1 teaspoon Old Bay seafood seasoning (in spice section)	

- In a microwave-safe bowl, microwave the stew vegetables for 3 minutes, stirring halfway through.
- In a large saucepan or Dutch oven, combine the soup, half-and-half, Old Bay seasoning, shrimp, crabmeat, and scallops. Cook over medium-low heat, stirring frequently to prevent scorching or burning.
- Once the vegetables are thoroughly cooked, stir them into the seafood mixture.
- Bring to a low boil. Serve when heated through, 10 to 15 minutes.

Yield: 8 (1-cup) servings

Calories: 331 (9% fat); Total Fat: 3 gm; Cholesterol: 151 mg; Carbohydrate: 42 gm; Dietary Fiber: 4 gm; Protein: 33 gm; Sodium: 1647 mg
Diabetic Exchanges: 2 starch, 2 vegetable, 3 very lean meat

Preparation time: 10 minutes
Cooking time: 20 minutes
Total time: 30 minutes or less

Menu Idea: This hearty stew is a meal in itself, so there is no need to serve anything with it. If you want a dessert, serve Rainbow Fresh Fruit Salad found on page 136 of this book.

Seafood Stew

My entire family likes this, but the shrimp and scallops make it an expensive dish. In my house it is a special treat. Thank goodness imitation crabmeat saves on cost.

1	(14-ounce) can 98% fat-free chicken broth	1	(14.5-ounce) can stewed tomatoes, undrained
1	teaspoon Old Bay seafood seasoning (in spice section)	1 1/2	pounds imitation crabmeat, cut into bite-size pieces
1	(29-ounce) can stew vegetables, undrained	1 1/2	pounds frozen scallops
		1	pound frozen cooked shrimp, shells and tails removed

- In a large saucepan or Dutch oven, combine the chicken broth, Old Bay seasoning, vegetables with juice, tomatoes with juice, crabmeat, and scallops. Cook over medium-high heat until the scallops are fully cooked, about 10 minutes. They will be opaque in color and tender when cooked.
- Stir in the shrimp. Once the broth comes to a low boil the soup is fully cooked and ready to eat. Turn off the heat. You do not want to overcook; otherwise the shrimp will become chewy and tough.
- If desired garnish with parsley flakes for added color.
- Serve immediately.

Yield: 12 (1-cup) servings

Calories: 199 (6% fat); Total Fat: 1 gm; Cholesterol: 120 mg; Carbohydrate: 18 gm; Dietary Fiber: 2 gm; Protein: 27 gm; Sodium: 646 mg
Diabetic Exchanges: 1 starch, 3 1/2 very lean meat

Preparation time: 5 minutes
Cooking time: 20 minutes
Total time: 25 minutes or less

Menu Ideas: For a complete meal serve with Garlic Crisps (page 29) from *Busy People's Down-Home Cooking Without the Down-Home Fat.* I also like having a side dish of Sassy Slaw (page 91) from *Busy People's Low-Fat Cookbook.*

Pork Stew

Here is another hometown favorite that many "heart-conscious" folks thought they could not eat, but I'm happy to say, "Enjoy!"

1 ½ pounds pork tenderloin, cut into bite-size pieces	2 (1-pound) bags vegetables for stew (I use Freshlike)
2 tablespoons minced garlic	2 (12-ounce) jars fat-free pork gravy (I use Heinz)
¾ teaspoon ground sage	¼ teaspoon ground black pepper
1 (14.5-ounce) can no-salt-added sliced stewed tomatoes	

Stove top Method:

- In a $4\frac{1}{2}$-quart nonstick saucepan over high heat, combine the tenderloin, garlic, sage, tomatoes, vegetables, gravy, and pepper. Bring to a full boil, stirring occasionally to prevent burning.
- Reduce the heat to medium. Continue boiling for 10 to 12 minutes or until the vegetables are tender, stirring occasionally.

Slow Cooker Method:

- Combine all the ingredients in a slow cooker. Stir until well mixed.
- Cover and cook on low for 8 to 9 hours or on high for 4 to 5 hours.

Yield: 9 (1-cup) servings

Calories: 193 (13% fat); Total Fat: 3 gm; Cholesterol: 51 mg; Carbohydrate: 22 gm; Dietary Fiber: 1 gm; Protein: 18 gm; Sodium: 487 mg
Diabetic Exchanges: 2 very lean meat, 1 starch, 1½ vegetable

Preparation time: 10 minutes
Cooking time: 15 minutes or less
Total time: 25 minutes or less

Menu Idea: It's a meal in itself, but if you'd like a green vegetable with it, I recommend the terrific flavors of the Tabbouleh Tossed Salad (page 61) from *Busy People's Down-Home Cooking Without the Down-Home Fat.*

Green Chilies Stew

My assistant, Brenda, tried this recipe with both beef and chicken. Her friends and family thought the stew was good prepared both ways.

2	pounds beef eye of round, cut into ¼-inch cubes	2	(4.5-ounce) cans chopped green chilies
2	medium onions, chopped	I	(14-ounce) can 99% fat-free beef broth (I use Swanson's)
I	(15-ounce) can pinto beans, drained and rinsed	2	teaspoons minced garlic
I	(14.5-ounce) can diced tomatoes, undrained		

- Brown the eye of round and onions in a nonstick skillet. Drain the fat.
- Coat a slow cooker with nonfat cooking spray. Add the browned meat and onions, pinto beans, tomatoes with juice, chilies, broth, and garlic.
- Stir until well mixed.
- Cook on high 7 to 8 hours or until the meat is tender.

Yield: 8 (1-cup) servings

Calories: 222 (18% fat); Total Fat: 4 gm; Cholesterol: 58 mg; Carbohydrate: 15 gm; Dietary Fiber: 5 gm; Protein: 29 gm; Sodium: 446 mg
Diabetic Exchanges: ½ starch, 1 ½ vegetable, 3 lean meat

Preparation time: 10 minutes

Menu Ideas: I like to eat this as it is, but some people like to serve it over brown rice. Southwestern Corn Bread (page 40) from *Busy People's Slow Cooker Cookbook* and a tossed salad make a nice meal.

Creamy Chili

Although the name of this recipe sounds outrageously fattening, have no fear! It is not. And every bite bursts with an explosion of flavor!

1 (12-ounce) bag Ground Meatless* crumbles or ³/4 pound ground eye of round, cooked	¹/4 teaspoon ground cinnamon
1 (15-ounce) can chili beans, undrained	1 (10³/4-ounce) can 98% fat-free cream of celery soup
1 (1.25-ounce) envelope chili seasoning mix, not prepared	2 (10³/4-ounce) cans water
	1 cup fat-free sour cream

- In a medium saucepan over medium heat, combine the Ground Meatless, chili beans, chili seasoning mix, cinnamon, soup, water, and sour cream and bring to a low boil, 4 to 5 minutes.
- Serve immediately.

Note: For a pretty serving presentation, sprinkle 1 tablespoon fat-free Cheddar cheese over each 1-cup serving. I like crumbling about 5 baked tortilla chips on top of each serving, also. *For more information on Ground Meatless see page 16.

Yield: 8 (1-cup) servings

(Nutritional information does not include Cheddar cheese or tortilla chips.)
(with Ground Meatless) Calories: 172 (10% fat); Total Fat: 2 gm; Cholesterol: 7 mg; Carbohydrate: 24 gm; Dietary Fiber: 5 gm; Protein: 15 gm; Sodium: 886 mg
Diabetic Exchanges: 1¹/2 starch, 1¹/2 very lean meat
(with ground eye of round) Calories: 194 (30% fat); Total Fat: 6 gm; Cholesterol: 31 mg; Carbohydrate: 20 gm; Dietary Fiber: 3 gm; Protein: 14 gm; Sodium: 768 mg
Diabetic Exchanges: 1¹/2 starch, 1¹/2 lean meat

Preparation time: 10 minutes
Cooking time: 5 minutes or less
Total time: 15 minutes or less

Menu Ideas: My family likes the Tomato Biscuits (page 59) along with a relish tray of assorted fresh vegetables and Buttermilk Salad Dressing (page 53) both from *Busy People's Low-Fat Cookbook.*

Strawberry & Vanilla Cream Cottage Cheese Salad

When I was about six years old I started mixing things together to create my own dishes. One of my favorites was mixing cottage cheese with jelly. My family thought I was crazy, but I didn't like cottage cheese by itself; however I loved it mixed with jelly.

1	cup fresh strawberries, sliced (about 6 large)	1/4	cup no-sugar-added strawberry preserves
3	plus 1 tablespoons Splenda Granular	1	teaspoon vanilla extract
2	cups fat-free cottage cheese		

- In a bowl, gently stir together the sliced strawberries and 1 tablespoon of the Splenda. Set aside.
- In a separate bowl, stir together the remaining 3 tablespoons Splenda, cottage cheese, strawberry preserves, and vanilla until well mixed.
- Gently stir the sweetened strawberries into the cottage cheese mixture.
- Eat immediately or keep refrigerated until ready to eat.

Note: You can substitute blueberries, peaches, or raspberries for the strawberries for just about 20 more calories. Be sure to substitute blueberry preserves, peach preserves, or raspberry preserves for the strawberry preserves as well. For the raspberries you will have to add 2 tablespoons of Splenda at the beginning.

Yield: 6 ($\frac{1}{2}$-cup) servings

Calories: 74 (0% fat); Total Fat: 0 gm; Cholesterol: 3 mg; Carbohydrate: 9 gm; Dietary Fiber: 1 gm; Protein: 10 gm; Sodium: 254 mg
Diabetic Exchanges: $\frac{1}{2}$ fruit, $1\frac{1}{2}$ very lean meat

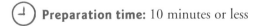 **Preparation time:** 10 minutes or less

Menu Ideas: This is a great, healthy lunch or snack combining fat-free protein (cottage cheese) with low-calorie carbohydrates (fruit). If you feel you need more to fill you up, enjoy fresh vegetable sticks with Vegetable Dip (page 48) from *Busy People's Low-Fat Cookbook* or a fresh garden salad with your favorite fat-free dressing.

Cherry Holiday Salad

This salad is great for the holidays with turkey or ham. It's slightly tart and tangy.

1 cup diet lemon-lime soda (7-Up or diet Sprite)	1 (11-ounce) can mandarin oranges
1 (.35-ounce) package sugar-free cherry gelatin (I use Royal)	¼ cup Equal Spoonful sweetener
1 (14.5-ounce) can pitted, tart, red cherries in water (I use Thank You brand)	1 (8-ounce) container fat-free whipped topping (I use Cool Whip)
	¼ cup finely chopped walnuts

- Heat the soda in the microwave on high for 1 minute.
- In a large bowl, briskly stir the gelatin into the soda, stirring until completely dissolved.
- Drain the juices from the cherries and mandarin oranges with juice into the gelatin. Stir until well mixed.
- On a dinner plate, smash the cherries with a potato masher.
- Sprinkle the sweetener over the smashed cherries and stir until well mixed.
- With a whisk, briskly stir the sweetened cherries, oranges, whipped topping, and walnuts into the gelatin until well mixed.
- Pour into a pretty glass serving bowl. Refrigerate until firm. (I like to make it the night before.)

Yield: 10 (½-cup) servings

Calories: 89 (21% fat); Total Fat: 2 gm; Cholesterol: 0 mg; Carbohydrate: 14 gm; Dietary Fiber: 1 gm; Protein: 1 gm; Sodium: 48 mg
Diabetic Exchanges: ½ fruit, ½ other carbohydrate

Preparation time: 10 minutes or less
Cooking time: 1 minute
Total time: 10 minutes or less plus time to set

Menu Idea: This tasty salad fits in perfectly as a dessert, too! Just think of how good it'll taste on Christmas or Thanksgiving after a turkey dinner!

Cinnamon & Spice
Cottage Cheese Salad

I created this unique recipe out of sheer necessity. I was in Texas taping a show for Life Today *with James and Betty Robison. I had a little refrigerator in my hotel room, so I stopped at a local grocery store before checking into the hotel to purchase a few things to eat. This combination hit the spot and was a sure winner! I will be making this again and again. I love the fact that it is so healthy also.*

1 cup fat-free cottage cheese	1 individual packet Splenda
1 (0.14-ounce) envelope instant sugar-free, low-calorie spiced cider drink mix, not prepared	

- In a bowl (or in my case I only had the cup provided by the hotel), stir together the cottage cheese, spiced cider mix, and Splenda until well mixed.
- Eat immediately or keep refrigerated until ready to eat.

Yield: 2 ($\frac{1}{2}$-cup) servings

Calories: 90 (0% fat); Total Fat: 0 gm; Cholesterol: 5 mg; Carbohydrate: 7 gm;
Dietary Fiber: 0 gm; Protein: 14 gm; Sodium: 395 mg
Diabetic Exchanges: $\frac{1}{2}$ other carbohydrate, 2 very lean meat

Preparation time: 2 minutes or less

Menu Ideas: I like to eat this for a quick "pick-me-up" snack. To make a light meal cut a piece of fresh fruit such as a small apple or a pear into it.

Fresh Fruit Salad

The vibrant color combination of this salad is beautiful! It's perfect for breakfast, instead of fruit juice.

1	cup cold water	4	clementines (or navel oranges), sliced into 1/3-inch rings and sectioned
1	tablespoon lemon juice		
3	medium bananas, cut into 1/2-inch slices	2	individual packets Splenda
1	pint fresh strawberries, cut into 1/3-inch slices		

- In a medium serving bowl, mix the cold water and lemon juice together.
- Add the banana slices to the lemon-water and soak for 4 minutes.
- Drain the bananas, discarding the lemon-water.
- Very gently stir the strawberries, clementine (or orange) sections, and Splenda into the bananas.
- Cover and keep chilled until ready to eat.

Yield: 10 ($\frac{1}{2}$-cup) servings

Calories: 68 (0% fat); Total Fat: 0 gm; Cholesterol: 0 mg; Carbohydrate: 17 gm; Dietary Fiber: 3 gm; Protein: 1 gm; Sodium: 1 mg
Diabetic Exchanges: 1 fruit

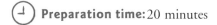 **Preparation time:** 20 minutes

Menu Ideas: Great for breakfast, brunch, or with fat-free cottage cheese for lunch. I really like this served with the Breakfast Pizza on page 86 of this book as well.

Rainbow Fresh Fruit Salad

This salad is most economical during the summer when the fruit is in season.

1 cup fresh blueberries	2 cups fresh strawberries
2 cups cubed honeydew melon	8 individual packets Splenda
2 cups cubed cantaloupe	

- Gently toss the blueberries, honeydew, cantaloupe, strawberries, and Splenda together until well mixed.
- Keep chilled until ready to serve.

Yield: 7 (1-cup) servings

Calories: 61 (0% fat); Total Fat: 0 gm; Cholesterol: 0 mg; Carbohydrate: 15 gm; Dietary Fiber: 2 gm; Protein: 1 gm; Sodium: 11 mg
Diabetic Exchanges: 1 fruit

 Preparation time: 30 minutes

 Menu Ideas: Breakfast and brunches are finished off nicely with a serving of this fruit salad to curb the sweet tooth. Try this recipe with the Citrus Pancakes (page 8) or the French Toast Sticks (page 7) both from *Busy People's Down-Home Cooking Without the Down-Home Fat.*

Fluffy Fruit Salad

Brenda Crosser from Florida says her grandmother gave this recipe to her years ago; of course her recipe was not sugar free or fat free. This one is just as good, and Brenda can still taste those homemade butter cookies her grandmother served with it.

1 (16-ounce) container fat-free cottage cheese	1 (0.3-ounce) sugar-free flavored gelatin (I use orange)
1 (8-ounce) container fat-free whipped topping (I use Cool Whip)	1 (15-ounce) can fruit cocktail in fruit juice, well drained (I use Del Monte Fruit Naturals)

■ In a bowl, stir the cottage cheese, whipped topping, gelatin, and fruit cocktail together until well mixed.

Yield: 10 (½-cup) servings

Calories: 86 (0% fat); Total Fat: 0 gm; Cholesterol: 2 mg; Carbohydrate: 13 gm; Dietary Fiber: 0 gm; Protein: 6 gm; Sodium: 179 mg
Diabetic Exchanges: 1 fruit, 1 very lean meat

Preparation time: 5 minutes or less

Menu Ideas: Brenda says her grandmother used to serve this with butter cookies for dessert. Since butter cookies are so high in sugar and fat, try the Apple Spice Cookies (page 220) or the Perfect Pineapple Cookies (page 224) both from *Busy People's Low-Fat Cookbook.*

Melon Salad

The green, orange, and red colors add cheer to any meal.

2	cups fresh honeydew melon, cubed	2	cups fresh watermelon, cubed
2	cups fresh cantaloupe, cubed	6	individual packets Splenda

- Gently toss the honeydew, cantaloupe, watermelon, and Splenda together until well mixed.
- Keep chilled until ready to serve.

Note: For faster preparation time you can buy the melons pre-cut, but beware, buying the melons pre-cut is expensive.

Yield: 6 (1-cup) servings

Calories: 58 (0% fat); Total Fat: 0 gm; Cholesterol: 0 mg; Carbohydrate: 14 gm; Dietary Fiber: 1 gm; Protein: 1 gm; Sodium: 11 mg
Diabetic Exchanges: 1 fruit

Preparation time: 30 minutes or less

Menu Ideas: This makes a perfect ending to heavy meals such as Beef & Rice Casserole (page 112) or Beef Tips & Angel Hair Pasta (page 113) both from *Busy People's Down-Home Cooking Without the Down-Home Fat.*

Reuben Salad

If you like Reuben sandwiches you'll like this.

4 cups chopped iceberg lettuce	1 (2.5-ounce) package lean, thinly sliced corned beef
1 (14-ounce) can sauerkraut, rinsed and squeezed dry	1/2 cup fat-free Thousand Island salad dressing
2 slices fat-free Swiss cheese, cut into pieces (I use Kraft)	1/2 cup rye croutons (fat-free are available)

- Toss the lettuce, sauerkraut, cheese, corned beef, salad dressing, and croutons together in a serving bowl.
- Serve immediately.

Note: Do not toss with dressing or croutons until time to eat. Otherwise the salad will get soggy.

Yield: 5 (1-cup) servings

Calories: 87 (13% fat); Total Fat: 1 gm; Cholesterol: 10 mg; Carbohydrate: 14 gm; Dietary Fiber: 3 gm; Protein: 5 gm; Sodium: 957 mg
Diabetic Exchanges: 1/2 very lean meat, 1/2 starch, 1 vegetable

Preparation time: 10 minutes

Menu Ideas: The Herb Chicken Cutlets on page 214 of this book and the Almost Homemade Dressing (page 76) from *Busy People's Down-Home Cooking Without the Down-Home Fat* are two dishes that will taste good with this salad for a complete meal.

Greek Salad

Greek condiments turn a boring tossed salad into something special.

1/4 teaspoon dried oregano	1/2 cup chopped onion (about 1 small onion)
1 (14.5-ounce) can no-salt-added diced tomatoes, drained (or 18 cherry tomatoes)	12 small, pitted black olives, cut into thin slices
1 cup fat-free red wine vinegar salad dressing (I use Kraft)	1/4 cup finely crumbled feta cheese (approximately 1 1/2 ounces)
2 (10-ounce) bags lettuce (I use Dole European Brand)	

- In a small bowl, mix together the oregano, tomatoes, and salad dressing until well mixed. Set aside and keep refrigerated until ready to eat.
- In a large serving bowl, toss the lettuce and onion together. Keep chilled until ready to serve.
- Just before serving, toss the salad with the salad dressing mixture until well coated.
- Top with the olives and sprinkle with the cheese. Serve chilled.

Note: Do not toss the lettuce with the salad dressing until ready to serve, as this will make your salad soggy.

Yield: 7 (2-cup) servings

Calories: 60 (29% fat); Total Fat: 2 gm; Cholesterol: 5 mg; Carbohydrate: 9 gm; Dietary Fiber: 2 gm; Protein: 2 gm; Sodium: 577 mg
Diabetic Exchanges: 2 vegetable, 1/2 fat

Preparation time: 10 minutes or less

Menu Ideas: This salad accompanies omelets wonderfully for brunches. Try the Breakfast Scramble on page 66 in this book. It also tastes great with Italian entrées like Chicken Fettuccine (page 152) from *Busy People's Low-Fat Cookbook.*

Spinach Orange Salad

It's pretty and light, and the combination is just right!

1 (10-ounce) package fresh spinach, stems removed if desired	1/2 cup fat-free sour cream (I use Breakstone)
1 (11-ounce) can mandarin oranges	2 tablespoons Splenda Granular
1/4 cup real bacon bits (I use Hormel)	1/2 cup fat-free croutons
	1/4 medium red onion, cut into 1/8-inch rings and separated

- Put the spinach in a large bowl and set aside.
- Drain the juice from the mandarin oranges into a medium bowl. Set the oranges aside.
- With a whisk, briskly mix the bacon bits, sour cream, and Splenda into the mandarin orange juice until well blended.
- Pour the dressing over the spinach and toss. Garnish with the orange segments, croutons, and onion.

Note: Do not toss the salad or croutons in the dressing until ready to serve, or the salad will become soggy.

Yield: 8 (1-cup) servings

Calories: 55 (16% fat); Total Fat: 1 gm; Cholesterol: 4 mg; Carbohydrate: 9 gm; Dietary Fiber: 1 gm; Protein: 4 gm; Sodium: 164 mg
Diabetic Exchanges: 1/2 fruit

Preparation time: 10 minutes or less

Menu Idea: This salad is delicious with any casserole, such as the Spicy Ricey Vegetarian Dinner (page 147) from *Busy People's Low-Fat Cookbook.*

World's Easiest Spinach Salad

The ingredients aren't so unique or creative, but the way I assemble this salad is definitely unique.

1/2 cup liquid egg substitute or 6 egg whites	1/4 cup reduced-fat real bacon bits
6 cups fresh spinach, rinsed and cleaned (you can buy it already washed)	1/4 cup reduced-fat shredded mozzarella cheese
	1/3 cup fat-free French salad dressing

- In a microwave-safe bowl, stir the liquid egg substitute or egg whites together until well mixed. Cook on high in the microwave for 60 to 90 seconds or until fully cooked. Once the eggs are fully cooked, break them up into tiny pieces.
- In a large salad bowl, toss together the spinach, bacon bits, and cheese.
- Stir several ice cubes into the cooked eggs and stir. Once the eggs are fully chilled, drain the melted water and remove any remaining ice cubes from the bowl.
- Add the eggs to the spinach. Pour the salad dressing on top and toss before serving.

Yield: 4 (1½-cup) servings

Calories: 98 (22% fat); Total Fat: 2 gm; Cholesterol: 7 mg; Carbohydrate: 10 gm; Dietary Fiber: 2 gm; Protein: 9 gm; Sodium: 575 mg
Diabetic Exchanges: 1/2 other carbohydrate, 1 lean meat

Preparation time: 5 minutes or less
Cooking time: 2 minutes or less
Total time: 7 minutes or less

Menu Ideas: This salad basically goes with any entrée. Two of my favorites are Tarragon Chicken and Potatoes (page 139) and Chicken Cobbler (page 127) both from *Busy People's Slow Cooker Cookbook.*

Popeye's Favorite Salad

Even Olive Oyl couldn't create a more delicious spinach salad than this one. The grilled onions on this salad are what make it so special.

1 large sweet white onion, cut into ½-inch slices	1 (10-ounce) bag fresh, washed, and ready to eat baby spinach
1 pound lean eye of round steaks, fat trimmed away	6 hard boiled egg whites, chopped
	Fat-free salad dressing

- Spray the onion slices on both sides with nonfat cooking spray. If desired, lightly sprinkle one side of each onion slice with salt.
- Over medium heat, grill the steaks and onion slices on an outdoor grill. Cook to the desired degree of doneness.
- Cut the cooked steaks into long thin strips. If desired, sprinkle lightly with garlic salt.
- Cut the grilled onion slices into quarters.
- Place the spinach in a large, pretty salad bowl. Top with the egg whites, grilled onions, and steak strips.
- Serve immediately with salad dressing on the side or keep chilled for later use. It's good with the steak and onions either hot off the grill or chilled.

Yield: 8 (1-cup) servings

Calories: 100 (19% fat); Total Fat: 2 gm; Cholesterol: 29 mg; Carbohydrate: 4 gm; Dietary Fiber: 1 gm; Protein: 16 gm; Sodium: 96 mg
Diabetic Exchanges: 2 very lean meat, 1 vegetable

Preparation time: 10 minutes or less
Cooking time: 10 minutes or less
Total time: 20 minutes or less

Menu Ideas: Two servings of this salad is a meal in itself, however, if you'd like serve it with Garlic Crisps (page 29) from *Busy People's Down-Home Cooking Without the Down-Home Fat* or Pinwheel Dinner Rolls (page 64) from *Busy People's Low-Fat Cookbook.*

Asparagus Salad

This salad is a taste of spring!

1 **pound fresh asparagus**	1 **teaspoon Splenda Granular**
³/4 cup fat-free red wine vinegar salad dressing	

- Cook the asparagus in boiling water for 5 minutes. Drain.
- Gently toss the asparagus with the dressing and Splenda.

Yield: 5 (¹/₂-cup) servings

Calories: 39 (0% fat); Total Fat: 0 gm; Cholesterol: 0 mg; Carbohydrate: 8 gm; Dietary Fiber: 2 gm; Protein: 2 gm; Sodium: 482 mg
Diabetic Exchanges: 1¹/₂ vegetable

Preparation time: 5 minutes
Cooking time: 5 minutes
Total time: 10 minutes

Menu Idea: This salad accompanies any lean grilled meat.

Hen & Eggs Tossed Salad

Served with a fat-free sweet dressing such as poppy seed or red French, this salad is absolutely delicious!

8 ounces cooked chicken breast, cut into tiny pieces	1/2 cup liquid egg substitute, scrambled* (I use Egg Beaters)
8 cups chopped romaine or iceberg lettuce or 2 (1-pound) bags	1/2 cup fat-free Parmesan- or garlic-flavored croutons

- Toss the chicken, lettuce, and egg substitute.
- Add the croutons and serve.

Note: To prepare the eggs quickly, cook in the microwave for 90 seconds. Scramble with a whisk after cooking. Put in the freezer for 2 to 3 minutes to chill. Do not add your dressing or croutons until ready to serve or the salad will get soggy!

Yield: 8 (1-cup) servings

(Nutritional information does not include salad dressing)
Calories: 65 (16% fat); Total Fat: 1 gm; Cholesterol: 24 mg; Carbohydrate: 2 gm;
Dietary Fiber: 1 gm; Protein: 11 gm; Sodium: 61 mg
Diabetic Exchanges: 1 1/2 very lean meat

Yield: 4 (2-cup) servings

(Nutritional information does not include salad dressing)
Calories: 129 (16% fat); Total Fat: 2 gm; Cholesterol: 48 mg; Carbohydrate: 4 gm;
Dietary Fiber: 2 gm; Protein: 22 gm; Sodium: 122 mg
Diabetic Exchanges: 3 very lean meat, 1 vegetable

Preparation time: 15 minutes

Menu Ideas: This salad is great as a meal in itself for lunch. For dinner, serve with Sautéed Scallops with Garlic on page 180 of this book and Peppered Potato Salad (page 105) from *Busy People's Low-Fat Cookbook.*

Romaine & Pear Tossed Salad

I got this salad idea from a fancy restaurant. To be honest, my version is a lot tastier and a great deal less fattening! The flavorful and unique ingredient combination makes this out-of-the-ordinary salad perfect for special occasions.

6 cups fresh romaine lettuce, torn into bite-size pieces	1 medium fresh pear, cut into tiny pieces (about 1 cup)
1/4 cup reduced-fat real bacon bits	1/4 cup fat-free poppy seed salad dressing
1/4 cup blue cheese crumbles or feta cheese crumbles	2 individual packets Splenda

- In a large salad bowl, gently toss together the lettuce, bacon bits, cheese, pear, salad dressing, and Splenda.
- Keep chilled until ready to serve.

Note: If not serving the salad within 30 minutes, wait until right before serving to toss in the salad dressing and Splenda.

Yield: 4 (1½-cup) servings

Calories: 121 (32% fat); Total Fat: 4 gm; Cholesterol: 11 mg; Carbohydrate: 14 gm; Dietary Fiber: 3 gm; Protein: 6 gm; Sodium: 539 mg
Diabetic Exchanges: ½ fruit, ½ other carbohydrate, 1 medium-fat meat

Preparation time: 10 minutes or less

Menu Ideas: This tastes so good with the Orange Roughy with Seasoned Crumb Topping recipe on page 182 in this book along with the Tomato Biscuits (page 59) from *Busy People's Low-Fat Cookbook*.

Greek Pasta Salad

You will not believe how good this tastes!

16 ounces of your favorite pasta, cooked	1 large tomato, cut into ½-inch cubes
1½ cups fat-free red wine vinegar salad dressing (I use Kraft)	12 medium pitted black olives, sliced into thirds
1 (7-ounce) package tabbouleh (I use Oasis brand)	1 large cucumber, cut into tiny pieces
1 ounce feta cheese, finely crumbled	

- In a large bowl, combine the pasta, salad dressing, tabbouleh, cheese, tomato, black olives, and cucumber together. Keep chilled until ready to serve.

Note: For faster preparation, you can use leftover pasta from a previous meal. Just store it in cold water in the refrigerator. When ready to prepare the salad, drain the water and combine the pasta with the salad ingredients.

Yield: 14 (½-cup) servings

Calories: 200 (8% fat); Total Fat: 2 gm; Cholesterol: 2 mg; Carbohydrate: 39 gm; Dietary Fiber: 2 gm; Protein: 6 gm; Sodium: 404 mg
Diabetic Exchanges: 2½ starch

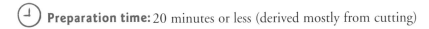 **Preparation time:** 20 minutes or less (derived mostly from cutting)

Menu Ideas: The Orange Roughy (page 151) from *Busy People's Low-Fat Cookbook* along with the Creamy Cucumbers (page 50) from *Busy People's Down-Home Cooking Without the Down-Home Fat* complete this as a meal.

Cucumber Salad with Bacon & Blue Cheese

The name of this recipe sounds as if this salad could be heavy and tossed in a cream-based dressing, but it is not. It is light and in a vinaigrette-based dressing. The longer it marinates the better it tastes.

3 large cucumbers, seeded and cut into 1/4- to 1/2-inch slices	1/4 cup crumbled blue cheese
1/4 cup reduced-fat real bacon bits	1/2 cup fat-free Italian salad dressing

- In a serving bowl, toss the cucumbers, bacon bits, cheese, and salad dressing together until well mixed.
- Serve chilled.

Yield: 8 (1-cup) servings

Calories: 60 (33% fat); Total Fat: 2 gm; Cholesterol: 6 mg; Carbohydrate: 7 gm; Dietary Fiber: 1 gm; Protein: 3 gm; Sodium: 326 mg
Diabetic Exchanges: 1/2 other carbohydrate, 1/2 fat

Preparation time: 15 minutes or less

Menu Idea: Tarragon Chicken and Potatoes (page 139) from *Busy People's Slow Cooker Cookbook* is great served with these cucumbers for a well-balanced meal.

Bacon & Blue Cheese Dressing

It is amazing that a salad dressing with both bacon and blue cheese can be made low fat and low calorie and still taste so terrific!

1 **(3-ounce) jar reduced-fat real bacon bits**	1/2 **cup buttermilk**
2 **cups fat-free sour cream**	1 **(0.59-ounce) envelope fat-free Ranch dip mix (I use Hidden Valley)**
1/2 **cup crumbled blue cheese**	

- In a bowl, stir the bacon bits, sour cream, blue cheese, buttermilk, and Ranch dip mix together until well mixed.
- Keep chilled until ready to serve.

Yield: 20 (2-tablespoon) servings

Calories: 63 (31% fat); Total Fat: 2 gm; Cholesterol: 10 mg; Carbohydrate: 5 gm; Dietary Fiber: 0 gm; Protein: 4 gm; Sodium: 305 mg
Diabetic Exchanges: 1/2 other carbohydrate, 1/2 fat

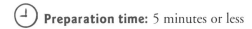 **Preparation time:** 5 minutes or less

Menu Ideas: Serve this dressing with fresh green lettuce for a salad friends will always remember. Try it on a salad served with entrées such as Cheesy Tuna Casserole (page 88) or Hamburger Gravy (page 107) both from *Busy People's Down-Home Cooking Without the Down-Home Fat.*

Ranch-Style Blue Cheese Salad Dressing

I got this fabulous tasting recipe idea from the country club restaurant where my daughter works. I loved theirs so much that I had to create my own low-calorie version, which is every bit as good, but a lot lower in fat and calories.

1 (0.59-ounce) envelope fat-free Ranch dip mix (I use Hidden Valley)	2 cups fat-free sour cream 1/2 cup skim milk 1/2 cup crumbled blue cheese

- In a bowl, combine the Ranch dip mix, sour cream, milk, and cheese together.
- Chill 1 to 24 hours before serving.

Yield: 20 (2-tablespoon) servings

Calories: 44 (22% fat); Total Fat: 1 gm; Cholesterol: 7 mg; Carbohydrate: 5 gm; Dietary Fiber: 0 gm; Protein: 3 gm; Sodium: 150 mg
Diabetic Exchanges: 1/2 other carbohydrate

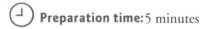 **Preparation time:** 5 minutes

Menu Ideas: This tastes terrific on any blend of fresh salad greens or as a dip for fresh vegetables. I recommend serving it with a mild-flavored entrée such as Macaroni and Cheese (page 87) or Steak on a Stick (page 120) both from *Busy People's Down-Home Cooking Without the Down-Home Fat.*

Blushing & Freckled Hens (Chicken Salad Spread)

The unique name of this recipe came from the color of the spread (light purple). The freckles come from the poppy seeds. My fellow First Place classmates gave this spread two thumbs up and said it should for sure be included in this book because of its great taste.

I (13-ounce) can chicken breast, drained	I tablespoon horseradish
	I teaspoon poppy seeds
1/3 cup jellied cranberry sauce	1/2 cup chopped onion

- In a medium bowl, stir together the chicken, cranberry sauce, horseradish, poppy seeds, and onion until well blended.
- Eat as is or keep chilled until ready to serve.

Yield: 4 (¼-cup) servings

Calories: 140 (13% fat); Total Fat: 2 gm; Cholesterol: 39 mg; Carbohydrate: 11 gm; Dietary Fiber: 1 gm; Protein: 18 gm; Sodium: 377 mg
Diabetic Exchanges: ½ other carbohydrate, 2½ very lean meat

Yield: 8 (2-tablespoon) servings

Calories: 70 (13% fat); Total Fat: 1 gm; Cholesterol: 20 mg; Carbohydrate: 6 gm; Dietary Fiber: 0 gm; Protein: 9 gm; Sodium: 188 mg
Diabetic Exchanges: ½ other carbohydrate, 1 very lean meat

Preparation time: 5 minutes

Menu Ideas: Serve on low-fat or fat-free crackers for a sweet and salty winning snack combination. As an appetizer this could also be spread on thin slices of dried bagel chips. Or spread this on lightly toasted bread for a tasty sandwich.

Pizza Pasta Salad

Serve this as a side dish for cookouts and picnics. It is also good as a main dish.

1 pound tri-colored spiral pasta	1 bunch green onions, chopped
1 (14-ounce) jar pizza sauce (I use Ragú)	2 ounces pepperoni, cut into tiny strips
1 (8-ounce) package fat-free shredded mozzarella cheese (I use Kraft)	$^3/_4$ cup fat-free red wine vinegar salad dressing (I use Seven Seas)

- Cook the pasta in boiling water as directed on the box, about 10 minutes. Rinse in cold water until chilled. Drain well.
- In a large bowl, combine the pasta, pizza sauce, cheese, green onions, pepperoni, and salad dressing and mix well.
- Serve as is or chill until ready to serve.

Yield: 18 ($^1/_2$-cup) servings

Calories: 143 (13% fat); Total Fat: 2 gm; Cholesterol: 5 mg; Carbohydrate: 22 gm; Dietary Fiber: 1 gm; Protein: 8 gm; Sodium: 404 mg
Diabetic Exchanges: $^1/_2$ very lean meat, 1$^1/_2$ starch

Yield: 9 (1-cup) servings

Calories: 285 (13% fat); Total Fat: 4 gm; Cholesterol: 9 mg; Carbohydrate: 44 gm; Dietary Fiber: 2 gm; Protein: 16 gm; Sodium: 808 mg
Diabetic Exchanges: 1 very lean meat, 3 starch

Preparation time: 5 minutes
Cooking time: 10 minutes
Total time: 15 minutes

Menu Idea: For a complete meal, serve with fresh green veggies (such as green peppers, celery sticks, or cucumber slices) and fat-free Buttermilk Ranch Dressing (page 53) from *Busy People's Low-Fat Cookbook* as a dip for the vegetables.

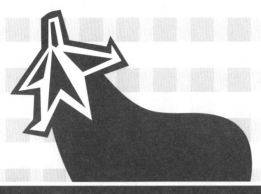

Simply Delicious
Side Dishes

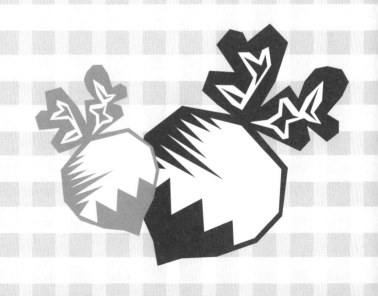

Sour Cream & Chives Mashed Potatoes

No one would believe that these light and fluffy potatoes aren't made from scratch.

2²/3 cups fat-free reduced-sodium chicken broth (or made from bouillon)	I (I5-ounce) can whole potatoes, drained
²/3 cup fat-free half-and-half	³/4 cup fat-free sour cream (I use Breakstone)
2²/3 cups instant potatoes (I use Betty Crocker Potato Buds)	¹/2 cup chopped fresh chives (or ¹/4 cup dried), divided

- In a 2-quart saucepan, bring the chicken broth and half-and-half to a full boil. Turn off the heat.
- Stir in the instant potatoes until moistened. Let sit for 30 seconds or until all the liquid is absorbed.
- In a microwave-safe bowl, mash the whole potatoes into tiny chunks. Microwave the potato chunks for up to 2 minutes or until fully heated.
- Combine the instant potatoes, warmed potato chunks, sour cream, and all but 1 teaspoon of the chives together in a serving bowl until well blended.
- Sprinkle the reserved 1 teaspoon chives on top.

Note: For a nice flavorful addition sprinkle ¼ cup real bacon bits on top. (I use Hormel.)

Yield: 10 (½-cup) servings

Calories: 100 (0% fat); Total Fat: 0 gm; Cholesterol: 2 mg; Carbohydrate: 20 gm; Dietary Fiber: 2 gm; Protein: 5 gm; Sodium: 255 mg
Diabetic Exchanges: 1½ starch
(with bacon bits) Calories: 110 (6% fat); Total Fat: 1 gm; Cholesterol: 4 mg; Carbohydrate: 20 gm; Dietary Fiber: 2 gm; Protein: 6 gm; Sodium: 344 mg
Diabetic Exchanges: 1½ starch

Preparation time: 10 minutes
Cooking time: 10 minutes
Total time: 20 minutes

Menu Idea: Serve with Chicken Fried Steak on page 204 of this book or baked chicken.

Creamy Dill Potatoes

The cream and herbs blended together enhance the potato flavor. Using frozen hash browns saves me oodles of time peeling, cutting, and chopping. And if you don't tell, no one will know you didn't start completely from scratch.

1 pound frozen southern-style hash browns (diced potatoes)	**1 tablespoon Ranch salad dressing mix, dry**
1 cup fat-free sour cream	**$^1/_8$ to $^1/_4$ teaspoon dried dill**

- In a microwavable bowl covered with wax paper microwave the hash browns for 3 minutes. Do not add water.
- Stir, cover, and continue microwaving for another 3 to 4 minutes or until the potatoes are piping hot and tender.
- In a bowl combine the sour cream, Ranch salad dressing mix, and dill and stir until well blended.
- Add the potatoes and gently stir until they are evenly coated.
- Serve immediately.

Yield: 4 ($^1/_2$-cup) servings

Calories: 167 (0% fat); Total Fat: 0 gm; Cholesterol: 10 mg; Carbohydrate: 35 gm; Dietary Fiber: 3 grams; Protein: 7 gm; Sodium: 358 mg
Diabetic Exchanges: 2 $^1/_2$ starch

Preparation time: 3 minutes or less
Cooking time: 7 minutes or less
Total time: 10 minutes or less

Menu Idea: These are great with the Orange Roughy (page 151) from *Busy People's Low-Fat Cookbook* along with a fresh tossed salad topped with your favorite fat-free salad dressing.

Parmesan Potatoes

Here's a quick and easy way to perk up your French fries.

3   tablespoons grated fat-free Parmesan cheese
$^{1}/_{2}$ teaspoon black pepper
1   teaspoon garlic salt

1   (1-pound) package frozen French fries (I use Flavorite brand)
Nonfat butter-flavored cooking spray

- Preheat the oven to 450 degrees. Coat a baking sheet with nonfat cooking spray.
- Combine the cheese, pepper, and garlic salt in a large plastic zip-top bag. Shake until well mixed.
- Add the French fries to the bag with seasonings. Shake until well coated.
- Pour the entire contents of the bag onto the prepared baking sheet. Spray the seasoned fries with cooking spray.
- Bake for 20 minutes or until golden brown.

Yield: 4 servings

Calories: 111 (6% fat); Total Fat: 1 gm; Cholesterol: 0 mg; Carbohydrate: 24 gm; Dietary Fiber: 2 gm; Protein: 3 gm; Sodium: 562 mg
Diabetic Exchanges: 1$^{1}/_{2}$ starch

Preparation time: 5 minutes
Cooking time: 20 minutes
Total time: 25 minutes

Menu Idea: These go well with fat-free hot dogs, lean steak, or chicken breasts.

Sweet Potato Silver Dollar Pancakes

These melt in your mouth and are so yummy that it was difficult for me not to eat more than I should.

1 (40-ounce) can yams in syrup, drained	3 individual packets Splenda
1/2 cup egg substitute (I use Egg Beaters) or 4 egg whites, beaten lightly	1/2 tablespoon molasses (optional)
	3 tablespoons light butter or light margarine*
1/3 cup reduced-fat all-purpose baking mix (Bisquick)	Light salt (optional)

- Preheat a skillet on high while mixing the ingredients.
- In a medium-size mixing bowl beat the yams, egg, baking mix, Splenda, and molasses (if desired) with electric mixer until well blended, 1 to 2 minutes. Some lumps are okay.
- Melt 1 tablespoon of the light butter or margarine in the skillet, covering the entire skillet surface.
- Put 1 tablespoon of the sweet potato mixture in the skillet.
- Repeat until the skillet is full of mini-pancakes. (I cooked four rows of three, for a total of twelve at one time.)
- Once all of your mini-pancakes are on the skillet, coat the tops of them with nonfat cooking spray. Press the mini-pancakes down until they are flat, about ¼ inch to ⅓ inch thick.
- Cook on high for 2 to 3 minutes per side or until the bottoms are toasty brown, not light brown.
- Turn the mini-pancakes over and continue cooking for another 2 to 3 minutes or until toasty brown on the other side. Do not spray a second time.

- Place the cooked sweet potato pancakes on a plate and lightly sprinkle with salt, if desired.
- Do not stack the pancakes unless you have a sheet of wax paper between each layer. The recipe will make about thirty-six 1½-inches in diameter pancakes.

Note: I use Smart Balance because it has half the fat of butter or margarine and it has no trans fats.

Yield: 12 servings (3 mini-pancakes per serving)

Calories: 97 (15% fat); Total Fat: 2 gm; Cholesterol: 0 mg; Carbohydrate: 19 gm; Dietary Fiber: 2 gm; Protein: 2 gm; Sodium: 118 mg
Diabetic Exchanges: 1 starch

Preparation time: 5 minutes or less
Cooking time: 6 minutes per every dozen
Total time: 25 minutes or less

Menu Idea: Don't mistake these for light, fluffy traditional pancakes. These are like mini mashed sweet potato disks lightly fried. They are excellent with lean ham or pork tenderloin. They also taste great for brunch or lunch with omelets or frittatas. Try them with the Mushroom & Onion Frittata (page 91) from *Busy People's Down-Home Cooking Without the Down-Home Fat.*

Sweet Potato Sticks

These are a favorite for everyone in our family. Although they're not crispy like French fries, they're definitely delicious!

I large sweet potato	Light salt

- Preheat the oven to 425 degrees. Spray two baking sheets with nonfat cooking spray.
- Scrub the sweet potato and cut into ¼-inch-thick slices about 3 inches long.
- Arrange the potato sticks on the prepared baking sheets. Spray the potato slices with nonfat cooking spray.
- Bake for 10 minutes, or until the bottoms are slightly brown. (Baking time will depend on the thickness of the fries.)
- Turn over. Spray again with nonfat cooking spray. Bake an additional 7 to 10 minutes or until the potatoes are tender.
- Sprinkle lightly with salt. Serve hot.

Note: For sweet potato disks cut the potato into thin round slices like you would if you were making potato chips.

Yield: 3 servings

Calories: 95 (0% fat); Total Fat: 0 gm; Cholesterol: 0 mg; Carbohydrate: 24 gm; Dietary Fiber: 3 gm; Protein: 2 gm; Sodium: 33 mg
Diabetic Exchanges: 1½ starch

Preparation time: 5 minutes or less
Cooking time: 20 minutes or less
Total time: 25 minutes or less

Menu Idea: These are great with sandwiches or fat-free hot dogs.

Potato Puffs

These potatoes are uniquely different!

¹/₂ teaspoon garlic powder	1 (5-ounce) can white chicken in water (I used Swanson), undrained
1³/₄ cups fat-free chicken broth	
1¹/₂ cups dry instant mashed potatoes	1 cup seasoned home fries, thawed (I use Bob Evans)
¹/₂ cup liquid egg substitute (or 4 egg whites, beaten)	2 tablespoons light margarine (I use Ultra Light Promise)

- Preheat the oven to 400 degrees. Line two baking sheets with aluminum foil. Coat the foil with nonfat cooking spray.
- In a bowl, combine the garlic powder, chicken broth, instant potatoes, egg substitute, chicken, home fries, and margarine. Stir until well blended.
- Drop by rounded tablespoonfuls onto the prepared baking sheets.
- Bake for 12 to 14 minutes or until slightly brown on the edges.
- If desired, sprinkle with chopped fresh chives and serve with fat-free chicken gravy.

Note: For Ham Puffs just substitute 5 ounces of chopped, cooked ham for the chicken.

Yield: 12 (2-puff) servings

(with chicken) Calories: 130 (5% fat); Total Fat: 1 gm; Cholesterol: 5 mg; Carbohydrate: 25 gm; Dietary Fiber: 2 gm; Protein: 6 gm; Sodium: 164 mg
Diabetic Exchanges: ¹/₂ very lean meat, 1¹/₂ starch
(with ham) Calories: 133 (7% fat); Total Fat: 1 gm; Cholesterol: 5 mg; Carbohydrate: 25 gm; Dietary Fiber: 2 gm; Protein: 6 gm; Sodium: 262 mg
Diabetic Exchanges: ¹/₂ very lean meat, 1¹/₂ starch

Preparation time: 10 minutes
Cooking time: 12 minutes or less
Total time: 22 minutes or less

Menu Ideas: Great for brunch buffets, with omelets, or with egg-based entrées.

Unfried Veggies

My arteries and waistline know I can't eat fried foods. I never miss the fat or the mess with these crispy unfried veggies.

1 cup instant potatoes	4 egg whites
1/3 cup nonfat grated Parmesan cheese (I use Kraft Free)	4 to 5 cups bite-size fresh vegetables (mushrooms, onions, and zucchini)
3/4 teaspoon garlic salt	

- Preheat the oven to 400 degrees. Coat a baking sheet with nonfat cooking spray. If desired, line the baking sheet with aluminum foil and coat with cooking spray for faster cleanup.
- Mix the potatoes, Parmesan cheese, and garlic salt together in a small bowl.
- In a separate bowl beat the egg whites with a fork for one minute.
- Dip the vegetables, one at a time, into the beaten egg whites. Then dip into the dry mixture, coating well.
- Place on the prepared baking sheet, making sure the vegetables do not touch each other. Spray the vegetables lightly with nonfat cooking spray.
- Bake for 10 minutes. Turn over and bake an additional 5 minutes or until crispy and golden brown.
- Season with light salt, if desired. Serve hot.

Yield: 8 servings

Calories: 46 (0% fat); Total Fat: 0 gm; Cholesterol: 0 mg; Carbohydrate: 9 gm; Dietary Fiber: 1 gm; Protein: 3 gm; Sodium: 189 mg
Diabetic Exchanges: 2 vegetable

Preparation time: 15 minutes or less
Cooking time: 15 minutes
Total time: 30 minutes or less

Menu Idea: Serve with Crunchy Vegetable Spread on page 109 of this book for dipping.

Broccoli, Mushrooms & Onion

The flavor combinations from the vegetables complement and enhance each other.

6 cups fresh broccoli florets (tops only, about 1- to 1 1/2-inch pieces)	1/2 medium red onion, sliced and separated into rings
1 cup sliced fresh mushrooms	1/4 cup reduced-fat real bacon bits Butter-flavored spray

- Put a half inch of water in the bottom of a medium saucepan.
- Place the broccoli, mushrooms, and onion in the saucepan. Bring to a boil.
- Cover and cook on high for 2 minutes. Turn off the heat.
- Let sit, covered, for 10 to 15 minutes or until the broccoli is tender; drain.
- Sprinkle the bacon bits on top and spray with about 20 squirts of the butter spray.

Yield: 4 (1-cup) servings

Calories: 72 (23% fat); Total Fat: 2 gm; Cholesterol: 5 mg; Carbohydrate: 8 gm;
Dietary Fiber: 4 gm; Protein: 7 gm; Sodium: 280 mg
Diabetic Exchanges: 1 1/2 vegetable, 1/2 lean meat

Preparation time: 5 minutes or less
Cooking time: 17 minutes or less
Total time: 22 minutes or less

Menu Idea: This vegetable side dish goes great with home-style foods such as the Quick Fix Steak (page 97) or the Marinated Grilled Chicken Breast (page 105) both from *Busy People's Down-Home Cooking Without the Down-Home Fat.*

Sweet & Flavorful Cooked Onions

Just thinking about these superb, ever-so-lightly-sweetened, flavorful onions makes my mouth water. These taste wonderful.

2	medium Vidalia onions, cut in half, peeled, and sliced thin	1/4	cup fat-free Italian salad dressing
I	tablespoon water	I	individual packet Splenda

- In a 12-inch nonstick skillet separate the onions into rings. Cook the onions in the water, covered, over medium heat for 15 minutes, stirring once every 5 minutes. (Keep the lid on when not stirring to let them steam.)
- Meanwhile, in a small bowl combine the Italian salad dressing and Splenda and stir until the Splenda is completely dissolved and well mixed. Set aside.
- Once the onions are completely cooked turn off the heat and stir in the sweetened Italian dressing.
- Serve immediately while the onions are nice and hot.

Yield: 4 (1/2-cup) servings

Calories: 41 (0% fat); Total Fat: 0 gm; Cholesterol: 0 mg; Carbohydrate: 9 gm; Dietary Fiber: 2 gm; Protein: 1 gm; Sodium: 217 mg
Diabetic Exchanges: 2 vegetable

Preparation time: 5 minutes or less
Cooking time: 15 minutes
Total time: 20 minutes or less (and worth every moment!)

Menu Idea: I think these taste terrific on any plain ol' boring meat such as fat-free hot dogs, lean hamburgers, grilled chicken, or steak.

Freckled Sweetened Cooked Carrots

Children like the fun name of this recipe and when carrots are this yummy young ones ask for more. (The freckles are poppy seeds.)

1 teaspoon vanilla extract	1 tablespoon fat-free poppy seed salad dressing
1/4 cup Splenda Granular	
1 (1 pound) bag peeled mini carrots	

- Fill a medium-size saucepan with 1 inch of water.
- Stir the vanilla and Splenda into the water until dissolved.
- Add the carrots.
- Cover and cook on high for 10 minutes. (Steam will come out from under the lid. That is okay.)
- Drain all the water and gently stir in the poppy seed salad dressing until all of the carrots are evenly coated.
- Serve hot.

Yield: 6 ($\frac{1}{2}$-cup) servings

Calories: 39 (0% fat); Total Fat: 0 gm; Cholesterol: 0 mg; Carbohydrate: 8 gm; Dietary Fiber: 1 gm; Protein: 1 gm; Sodium: 52 mg
Diabetic Exchanges: 1$\frac{1}{2}$ vegetable

Preparation time: 2 to 3 minutes
Cooking time: 10 minutes
Total time: 13 minutes or less

Menu Idea: Quick Fix Steak (page 97) from *Busy People's Down-Home Cooking Without the Down-Home Fat* is mighty fine with these carrots and the Tomato Zing Salad on page 52 of the same cookbook.

Sautéed Mushrooms

I can't believe I haven't included these in one of my other cookbooks already. They are so delicious!

1 **pound mushrooms (I use the traditional button mushroom)**	1 **tablespoon low-sodium soy sauce**
1 **tablespoon Worcestershire sauce**	1 **tablespoon butter-flavored sprinkles, dry**
	Dash garlic salt

- Rinse the mushrooms and cut off the ends of the stems.
- Coat a 12-inch nonstick skillet with butter-flavored nonfat cooking spray and place over medium heat.
- Add the Worcestershire sauce and soy sauce.
- Add the mushrooms. Cover and cook for 7 to 10 minutes or until mushrooms are tender when pierced with a fork. Turn off the heat.
- Drain the juice from the skillet into a small bowl.
- Stir in the butter-flavored sprinkles and the garlic salt. Mix until completely dissolved.
- Pour the juice over the mushrooms and stir until they are well seasoned.
- Serve with a slotted spoon.

Yield: 6 ($\frac{1}{2}$-cup) servings

Calories: 23 (0% fat); Total Fat: 0 gm; Cholesterol: 0 mg; Carbohydrate: 4 gm; Dietary Fiber: 1 gm; Protein: 3 gm; Sodium: 156 mg
Diabetic Exchanges: 1 vegetable

Preparation time: 2 or 3 minutes
Cooking time: 7 to 10 minutes
Total time: 13 minutes or less

Menu Idea: I love these with a great lean steak on the grill. Remember, though, one serving of steak should only be about the size of a deck of cards or the size of your palm. Also serve the Bacon, Lettuce, and Tomato Salad (page 96) and Garlic Red Skins (page 117) both from *Busy People's Low-Fat Cookbook.*

Broiled Tomatoes with Feta Cheese & Bacon

The sweetness of the grape tomatoes united with the rye, feta, and bacon give this an impressive presentation and first-class taste.

9	slices cocktail rye bread	2	tablespoons finely chopped real bacon bits
I	(16-ounce) container grape tomatoes	1/2	teaspoon dried basil
1/2	cup reduced fat finely crumbled feta cheese		

- Preheat the broiler.
- Coat a 9-inch square glass dish with butter-flavored nonfat cooking spray. Arrange the rye bread in the bottom of the dish (three rows of three). If the bread in the corner of the dish is too tight you can trim it to fit.
- Arrange the whole grape tomatoes on top of the bread.
- Sprinkle the feta cheese on top of the tomatoes. Sprinkle the bacon and basil on top. Place the dish 3 inches below the broiler.
- Broil for 4 to 5 minutes or until the top is brown.
- Let it sit for a couple of minutes before serving as the piping hot tomatoes can easily burn your mouth. Cut into 6 servings.

Note: Cherry tomatoes can be substituted, but they usually are not as sweet.

Yield: 6 servings

Calories: 87 (26% fat); Total Fat: 3 gm; Cholesterol: 6 mg; Carbohydrate: 11 gm; Dietary Fiber: 2 gm; Protein: 5 gm; Sodium: 337 mg
Diabetic Exchanges: 1/2 starch, 1/2 lean meat

Preparation time: 5 minutes or less
Cooking time: 4 to 5 minutes
Total time: 10 minutes or less

Menu Idea: While these are broiling prepare the Sautéed Scallops with Garlic on page 180 of this book. The gourmet mixture of lettuces in the Slaw Salad (page 54) from *Busy People's Down-Home Cooking Without the Down-Home Fat* will round this meal off nicely.

Southwestern Kidney Beans & Tomato Casserole

People who like the spicy flavors inspired by Mexican cultures will especially like this dish. It definitely awakens the taste buds in a delicious way!

1/4 cup chopped fresh green onion* (Use the entire onion and green top)	1 (10-ounce) can diced tomatoes with green chilies, drained
1/2 teaspoon chili powder	1/2 cup fat-free shredded Cheddar cheese
1 (15.5 ounce) can kidney beans, drained (light or dark red)	

- In a medium-size microwave-safe bowl combine the green onion, chili powder, kidney beans, and diced tomatoes and stir until well mixed.
- Sprinkle the cheese on top.
- Cover with wax paper. (This will make the cheese smooth and creamy when it is all done cooking because the cheese will absorb the moisture from the other ingredients.)
- Cook in the microwave on full power for 2 minutes.
- Serve while it is hot.

Note: A super, quick way to cut the onions is with scissors.

Yield: 5 (1/2-cup) servings

Calories: 115 (6% fat); Total Fat: 1 gm; Cholesterol: 2 mg; Carbohydrate: 17 gm; Dietary Fiber: 6 gm; Protein: 9 gm; Sodium: 515 mg
Diabetic Exchanges: 1 starch, 1 very lean meat

Preparation time: 5 minutes or less
Cooking time: 2 minutes
Total time: 7 minutes or less

Menu Idea: Instead of the same ol' refried beans serve this delectable side dish with any Mexican themed meal such as tacos made with extra lean beef.

Sweet & Sour Bell Pepper Medley

This colorful side dish is ready to eat once it is thoroughly heated; however, for a more intense flavor put all of the ingredients in a zip-top bag and marinate for up to two days.

1/2 cup apple cider vinegar	1 yellow bell pepper, chopped into 1/2-inch pieces
1/2 cup Splenda Granular	
1 green bell pepper, chopped into 1/2-inch pieces	1 orange bell pepper, chopped into 1/2-inch pieces
1 red bell pepper, chopped into 1/2-inch pieces	

- In a saucepan over high heat combine the vinegar, Splenda, and all the bell peppers.
- Once the ingredients come to a full boil, cover, and cook for just under 1 minute or until the peppers are tender.
- Remove the peppers with a slotted spoon. They should be tender and the vibrant colors enhanced.
- Serve immediately.

Note: For Sweet and Sour Bell Pepper Salad do not cook but serve chilled. Nutritional values remain the same.

Yield: 8 (½-cup) servings

Calories: 20 (0% fat); Total Fat: 0 gm; Cholesterol: 0 mg; Carbohydrate: 5 gm; Dietary Fiber: 1 gm; Protein: 1 gm; Sodium: 2 mg
Diabetic Exchanges: 1 vegetable

Preparation time: 15 minutes or less
Cooking time: 5 minutes or less
Total time: 20 minutes or less

Menu Idea: This side dish is so very low in calories. It is a great choice to eat with lean steak such as flank steak, eye of round, or pork tenderloin. It's also good with a serving of a low-fat carbohydrate such as Cheesy Potato and Broccoli Casserole (page 91) from *Busy People's Slow Cooker Cookbook.*

French-Style Simmered Green Beans

The flavor combination of the salty bacon bits and lightly sweetened vanilla yogurt along with the garlic and seasonings complement these beans so smoothly and naturally; it seems as if all of these ingredients were meant to be together.

1 (28-ounce) can French-style green beans, drained	2 tablespoons reduced-fat real bacon bits
1 tablespoon minced garlic (from a jar)	1 tablespoon imitation butter-flavored sprinkles
2 tablespoons imitation Cheddar cheese sprinkles (found in the spice section)	1/4 cup fat-free, sugar-free vanilla yogurt

- In a medium nonstick saucepan over medium heat, stir together the green beans, garlic, cheese, bacon bits, and butter-flavored sprinkles until well mixed.
- Bring to a boil, stirring occasionally.
- Once boiling, stir in the yogurt. Reduce the heat to medium-low. Cook for another 2 to 3 minutes or until fully heated. Serve immediately.

Yield: 6 (1/2-cup) servings

Calories: 40 (15% fat); Total Fat: 1 gm; Cholesterol: 2 mg; Carbohydrate: 6 gm; Dietary Fiber: 1 gm; Protein: 2 gm; Sodium: 585 mg
Diabetic Exchanges: 1 vegetable

Preparation time: 5 minutes or less
Cooking time: 8 minutes or less
Total time: 13 minutes or less

Menu Idea : I served this with the Sautéed Scallops with Garlic on page 180 of this book and Cheese Biscuits (page 63) from *Busy People's Low-Fat Cookbook.* Dinner was a huge hit!

Wilted Fresh Spinach with Herbs

I am not a big "cooked spinach" fan, but I sure did like this! The herbs enhance and complement the spinach. People who like spinach will love this!

1 tablespoon fat-free margarine	1/2 teaspoon dried basil
1/2 teaspoon lemon-pepper seasoning	1/2 teaspoon dried parsley
1/2 teaspoon dried thyme	1 (10-ounce) bag fresh cleaned spinach

- Heat the margarine in a 12-inch nonstick skillet over medium-high heat.
- Add the lemon-pepper, thyme, basil, and parsley. Stir until all the margarine is melted and the seasonings are well blended.
- Add the spinach and stir to mix with the seasonings.
- Cover the skillet with a lid and cook for 2 minutes. The moisture from the spinach is enough to steam the leaves, and they will become soft and wilted.
- Stir. Cover again and cook for 2 or 3 minutes longer or until the spinach is wilted yet still tender. Serve immediately.

Yield: 4 ($\frac{1}{2}$-cup cooked) servings

Calories: 19 (0% fat); Total Fat: 0 gm; Cholesterol: 0 mg; Carbohydrate: 3 gm; Dietary Fiber: 2 gm; Protein: 2 gm; Sodium: 119 mg
Diabetic Exchanges: Free

Preparation time: 5 minutes or less
Cooking time: 5 minutes or less
Total time: 10 minutes or less

Menu Idea: In *Busy People's Low-Fat Cookbook* the Christmas Chicken with Rice Dinner on page 185 or the Smothered Steak on page 193 enhance the flavors of this dish.

Seasoned Buttered Broccoli

I wanted a seasoning that would enhance the flavor of broccoli. I found just the right combination of spices, including basil, red pepper, black pepper, onions, garlic, salt, and paprika in one ingredient: Cajun seasoning. I was pleasantly surprised how this seasoning blend complemented the broccoli without overpowering it. I will definitely make it again and again.

1 pound frozen broccoli 1 tablespoon reduced-fat margarine (I use Smart Balance Light*)	1 teaspoon imitation butter-flavored sprinkles, dry 1¹/₂ teaspoons Cajun seasoning

- In a microwave-safe container heat the broccoli, covered, on high for 6 minutes in the microwave, stirring after 3 minutes.
- Gently stir in the margarine, butter sprinkles, and Cajun seasoning until evenly distributed throughout the broccoli. Serve immediately.

Note: Smart Balance is found in the butter section of your grocery store. Its patented blend is used to help improve cholesterol.

Yield: 5 (³/₄-cup) servings

Calories: 36 (28% fat); Total Fat: 1 gm; Cholesterol: 0 mg; Carbohydrate: 5 gm; Dietary Fiber: 3 gm; Protein: 3 gm; Sodium: 208 mg
Diabetic Exchanges: 1 vegetable

Preparation time: 5 minutes or less
Cooking time: 6 minutes
Total time: 11 minutes or less

Menu Idea: This delicious broccoli will taste great with any home-style entrée such as the Swiss Steak and Potatoes in *Busy People's Slow Cooker Cookbook* on page 159 or any Italian entrée such as Chicken Linguine on page 95 of *Busy People's Down-Home Cooking Without the Down-Home Fat.*

Roasted Portabella Mushroom Caps

These taste so fantastic! I love a good steak, but there are times when I wouldn't mind just eating these instead.

4 large portabella mushroom caps, rinsed well and patted dry	¹/₄ teaspoon dry imitation butter-flavored sprinkles
Nonfat butter or olive oil spray	¹/₄ teaspoon Lawry's seasoned salt

- Remove the bottom rack from the oven.
- Place aluminum foil on the bottom of the oven, making sure the foil does not touch the heating elements.
- Preheat the oven to 500 degrees.
- Spray both sides of the portabella mushroom caps with cooking spray.
- Place the mushrooms with tops facing up on the top rack of the oven.
- Cook for 5 minutes.
- Using tongs, turn over each mushroom. Spray the bottoms of the mushrooms once again with cooking spray.
- Cook an additional 5 minutes.
- Remove from the oven. Evenly sprinkle the butter sprinkles and seasoned salt over the mushroom caps.
- Let the mushrooms sit for 2 to 3 minutes before serving. Allowing the mushrooms to rest helps them retain more moisture and flavor once they are cut.

Yield: 4 (1-mushroom-cap) servings

Calories: 15 (0% fat); Total Fat: 0 gm; Cholesterol: 0 mg; Carbohydrate: 3 gm; Dietary Fiber: 1 gm; Protein: 1 gm; Sodium: 105 mg
Diabetic Exchanges: Free

Preparation time: 8 minutes or less
Cooking time: 10 minutes
Total time: 18 minutes or less

Menu Idea: These taste terrific with a great lean steak such as London broil.

Sweet & Sour Cabbage

Sweet and sour cabbage is a favorite side dish at Polish weddings and festivities such as Christmas and Easter. It is traditionally served with mashed potatoes and kielbasa. From scratch this dish takes hours to make as it simmers to obtain the blend of flavors. However, my creative and clever way is much faster and easier to prepare yet every bit as tasty.

2 pounds sauerkraut rinsed thoroughly and squeezed dry*	1 tablespoon apple cider vinegar
³/4 cup sugar-free pink lemonade	5 tablespoons Splenda Granular

- In a 12-inch nonstick skillet combine the sauerkraut, pink lemonade, vinegar, and Splenda and stir until well mixed.
- Cook over medium-low heat for 10 minutes or until completely heated.
- Serve immediately or keep warm in a slow cooker on low until ready to eat.

Note: Put the sauerkraut in a strainer, run cold water over it for a minute or two, then squeeze dry by pressing with your hands.

Yield: 6 (¹/₂-cup) servings

Calories: 38 (12% fat); Total Fat: 1 gm; Cholesterol: 0 mg; Carbohydrate: 8 gm; Dietary Fiber: 5 gm; Protein: 1 gm; Sodium: 1080 mg
Diabetic Exchanges: 1¹/₂ vegetable

Preparation time: 2 minutes or less
Cooking time: 10 minutes or less
Total time: 12 minutes or less

Menu Ideas: Potatoes à la Larry (page 77) from *Busy People's Down-Home Cooking Without the Down-Home Fat* and a low-fat kielbasa make this a favorite Polish dinner people will remember.

Thai Napa Cabbage

The exotic Thai herbs and spices (found in the peanut sauce) when cooked with the Napa Cabbage (which is normally thought of as Chinese food) create an exciting and robust flavor. The fact that it is fast and easy to prepare, along with being low in calories, is a bonus I love.

1 tablespoon peanut sauce (found in spice aisle or Chinese food aisle of store)	1/4 teaspoon garlic salt
	1/8 teaspoon ground cinnamon
6 cups fresh shredded Napa Cabbage (firmly packed cups)	2 individual packets Splenda

- In a 12-inch nonstick skillet cook the peanut sauce over medium heat until hot.
- While the sauce is heating, shred the cabbage with a chef's knife, or to save time, in a food processor.
- Add the shredded cabbage to the peanut sauce. Do not stir. Cover and cook on medium heat for 5 to 7 minutes or until the cabbage is tender.
- Add the garlic salt, ground cinnamon, and Splenda and stir until all the ingredients are well blended.
- Serve with a slotted spoon so any excess juices can drain.

Yield: 4 (1/2-cup) servings

Calories: 36 (27% fat); Total Fat: 1 gm; Cholesterol: 0 mg; Carbohydrate: 4 gm; Dietary Fiber: 2 gm; Protein: 2 gm; Sodium: 84 mg
Diabetic Exchanges: 1 vegetable

Preparation time: 5 minutes or less
Cooking time: 7 minutes or less
Total time: 12 minutes or less

Menu Idea: Great with simple, home-style entrées such as lean steak or pork. It is also good with Smothered Steak (page 156), Spiced Ham Steaks (page 177), or Cubed Steak with Mushroom Gravy & Potatoes (page 150) all from *Busy People's Slow Cooker Cookbook.*

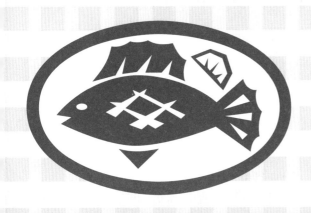

On the Go Entrées

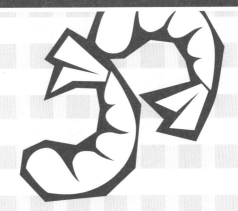

Oven-Fried Catfish

These babies are good!

1 (6.5-ounce) package cornbread mix (I use Gold Medal Smart Size)	1/2 cup liquid egg substitute (I use Egg Beaters)
1 cup all-purpose flour	1/2 cup skim milk
	2 pounds catfish fillets
	Garlic salt (optional)

- Preheat the oven to 450 degrees. Coat a baking sheet with nonfat cooking spray.
- In a shallow dish, mix the cornbread mix and flour together. Set aside.
- In a bowl mix the egg substitute and milk together.
- Dip the catfish into the flour mixture, then into the egg mixture, then again into the flour mixture.
- Coat the top of the fish with nonfat cooking spray.
- Place on the prepared baking sheets. Bake until the fish flakes easily when tested with a fork. (Allow 5 to 6 minutes for each 1/2 inch of thickness.)
- If desired, sprinkle lightly with garlic salt before serving.

Yield: 6 servings

Calories: 257 (21% fat); Total Fat: 6 gm; Cholesterol: 82 mg; Carbohydrate: 24 gm; Dietary Fiber: 2 gm; Protein: 25 gm; Sodium: 289 mg
Diabetic Exchanges: 4 very lean meat, 1$\frac{1}{2}$ starch

Preparation time: 5 minutes
Cooking time: 20 minutes or less
Total time: 25 minutes or less

Menu Idea: Like my old friend Earl from Tennessee would say, "Why, catfish never had it so good," when eaten with Sassy Slaw (page 91) from *Busy People's Low-Fat Cookbook* and Mama's Beans (page 71) from *Busy People's Down-Home Cooking Without the Down-Home Fat.*

Sautéed Scallops with Garlic

This extra-special entrée is pricey to prepare, so you may want to save it for an extra-special occasion. However, at the same time these scallops are so much less expensive to prepare at home compared to the high price you have to pay at a restaurant that this is a really good value, and the flavor is excellent!

1 1/2 pounds scallops (either bay or sea; frozen or fresh)

2 tablespoons light margarine (I use Smart Balance)

1 teaspoon minced garlic (from a jar)

1/4 teaspoon garlic salt

Juice of 1/2 medium fresh lemon

2 teaspoons dried chives or 1 tablespoon finely chopped fresh chives

- In a 12-inch nonstick skillet, combine the scallops, margarine, garlic, and garlic salt and cook over medium heat until the scallops are opaque, about 2 minutes per side for fresh 1-inch scallops or about 5 minutes per side for frozen.
- Once fully cooked, remove the scallops and place in a covered dish. Leave the liquid in the skillet.
- Add the lemon juice to the liquid in the skillet.
- Stir in the chives.
- Cook for about 1 to 2 minutes or until the liquid reduces to a glaze.
- Return the scallops to the skillet, stirring to coat the scallops with the sauce and to reheat the scallops, which will take 1 to 2 minutes longer.
- Serve immediately.

Yield: 6 (3-ounce) servings

Calories: 117 (20% fat); Total Fat: 3 gm; Cholesterol: 37 mg; Carbohydrate: 3 gm; Dietary Fiber: 0 gm; Protein: 19 gm; Sodium: 256 mg
Diabetic Exchanges: 3 very lean meat

Sautéed Shrimp:
Follow the recipe exactly except substitute shrimp for the scallops.

Calories: 102 (24% fat); Total Fat: 3 gm; Cholesterol: 168 mg; Carbohydrate: 1 gm;
Dietary Fiber: 0 gm; Protein: 18 gm; Sodium: 267 mg
Diabetic Exchanges: 3 very lean meat

Preparation time: 5 minutes or less
Cooking time: 10 minutes or less
Total time: 15 minutes or less

Menu Idea: This recipe is so low in calories that we can afford to splurge on higher calorie side dishes such as Twice Baked Potatoes (page 131) and Sassy Slaw (page 91) both from *Busy People's Low-Fat Cookbook.*

Orange Roughy with Seasoned Crumb Topping

You'll think you're cheating when eating this wonderful fish with its crumb topping that's flavored to perfection.

2 pounds frozen orange roughy fillets	1/2 teaspoon lemon pepper seasoning (found in spice section)
10 reduced-fat Ritz crackers	
1/2 teaspoon Old Bay seasoning (found in spice section)	1/2 tablespoon self-rising cornmeal mix

- Preheat the oven to 350 degrees.
- Line a jelly roll pan with aluminum foil.
- Place the fish fillets on the prepared pan and cover with foil. Bake for 8 minutes.
- Turn over the fish and bake for an additional 8 minutes.
- While the fish is baking, combine the crackers, Old Bay seasoning, lemon pepper, and cornmeal in a zip-top plastic bag.
- With a rolling pin or side of a can, gently hit the sealed bag to crush the crackers and then mix until well blended.
- Once the fish has cooked, remove it from the oven. Remove the foil.
- Increase the oven temperature to 400 degrees.
- Drain the cooking juices from the pan and sprinkle the seasoned crumbs evenly over the fish.
- Bake the fish on the top rack of the oven for another 8 minutes or until the fish is fully cooked. Serve immediately.

Note: The cooking time may vary depending on the thickness of the frozen fish. My fish was about 1/2 inch thick and the baking time is as directed. However, there were a few thin pieces of fish that baked more quickly. Check to see if the fish is fully cooked by inserting a fork in center of the thickest part of the fish. If it flakes easily and is white in color it is done. Do not overcook.

Yield: 8 (3-ounce cooked) servings

Calories: 95 (12% fat); Total Fat: 1 gm; Cholesterol: 23 mg; Carbohydrate: 3 gm;
Dietary Fiber: 0 gm; Protein: 17 gm; Sodium: 180 mg
Diabetic Exchanges: 3 very lean meat

Preparation time: 6 minutes or less
Cooking time: 24 minutes or less
Total time: 30 minutes or less

Menu Idea: This light, flaky fish tastes good with the Buttermilk
Biscuits on page 72 in this book and Green Beans and Potatoes (page
93) from *Busy People's Slow Cooker Cookbook.*

Creamy Shrimp & Bacon with Mushrooms

I got this idea from Chef Patrick at Louie P's Restaurant at Valleywood Golf Club where my daughter works. His was fantastic but way too high in calories for my daily caloric budget. So I created this and my family went nuts over it! I hope yours will, too.

3	cups cold skim milk	2 1/4	cups (about 8 ounces) sliced fresh mushrooms
3	tablespoons cornstarch	1 1/2	pounds jumbo (31 to 40 count) cooked shrimp (frozen is fine, but thaw before using)
2	teaspoons imitation butter flavoring (a liquid flavoring found in spices next to vanilla)		
1/2	cup reduced-fat real bacon bits	1/2	cup shredded Parmesan cheese

- In a 12-inch nonstick skillet, briskly mix together the milk, cornstarch, and butter flavoring using a whisk until the cornstarch is completely dissolved.
- Stir in the bacon and cook over medium heat for 5 to 10 minutes, stirring frequently to prevent lumps. The sauce will thicken as it cooks; the longer it cooks the thicker it will get. Be patient. You can't rush this process.
- When thickened, stir in the mushrooms. Cover and cook for 5 minutes, stirring frequently.
- Stir in the shrimp. Cover and cook for 3 to 5 minutes longer, stirring every couple of minutes.
- Add the cheese. Continue cooking, stirring continuously until the cheese is melted.
- Season with light salt or Mrs. Dash salt-free seasoning and pepper, if desired, before serving.

Yield: 6 (1-cup) servings

Calories: 249 (20% fat); Total Fat: 5 gm; Cholesterol: 235 mg; Carbohydrate: 11 gm; Dietary Fiber: 0 gm; Protein: 35 gm; Sodium: 766 mg
Diabetic Exchanges: 1 skim milk, 4 very lean meat

Preparation time: 10 minutes or less
Cooking time: 20 minutes or less
Total time: 30 minutes or less

Menu Idea: My family loves this served over cooked rainbow rotini pasta, which is spinach and tomato enriched macaroni product. I serve 1 cup of this over ½ cup of pasta per serving. I also serve steamed broccoli with it. Mmm!

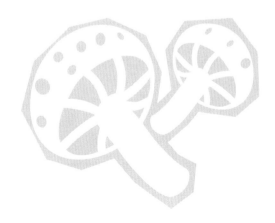

Crabby Fettuccine

Don't let the grouchy name of this recipe turn you away from a meal that will make you happy.

1 (12-ounce) box fettuccine, uncooked	1 teaspoon minced garlic
1 1/2 pounds imitation crab, cut into bite-size pieces	10 black olives, thinly sliced
1 (26-ounce) jar low-fat spaghetti sauce with mushrooms	1 teaspoon Splenda Granular
	Kraft Free grated Parmesan cheese (optional)

- Cook the pasta according to the package directions; drain.
- In a 12-inch nonstick skillet, cook the crab, spaghetti sauce, garlic, black olives, and Splenda over medium heat for 4 to 5 minutes or until completely heated.
- Serve over the hot pasta.
- If desired, sprinkle with Parmesan cheese.
- This dish is delicious reheated in the microwave. Simply stir the sauce in with the pasta and freeze or refrigerate until ready to use.

Yield: 8 (1-cup) servings

Calories: 302 (10% fat); Total Fat: 3 gm; Cholesterol: 17 mg; Carbohydrate: 50 gm; Dietary Fiber: 3 gm; Protein: 17 gm; Sodium: 1168 mg
Diabetic Exchanges: 3 starch, 1 vegetable, 1 1/2 very lean meat

Preparation time: 5 minutes or less
Cooking time: 15 minutes or less
Total time: 20 minutes or less

Menu Idea: For a fun Italian-themed meal serve with Green Beans Italiano (page 116) from *Busy People's Low-Fat Cookbook* and a tossed salad with fat-free Italian salad dressing.

Zany Ziti—One Pot Ziti

I like to take this creamy, zany, ziti dish to new moms. Usually they like it so much they want the recipe. It's so easy, and it becomes a family favorite.

2 1/4 cups water	1 (16-ounce) container fat-free sour cream (I use Land O Lakes)
2 (27.5-ounce) jars Ragú light pasta sauce	Kraft Free grated Parmesan cheese (optional)
1 (16-ounce) package ziti (I use Mueller's)	

- In a 4-quart nonstick Dutch oven or nonstick soup pot, bring the water and pasta sauce to a full boil over medium-high heat.
- Add the ziti. Stir until well mixed. Return to a full boil over medium-high heat.
- Reduce the heat to medium low. Cover and bring to a low boil.
- Cook for 25 minutes, stirring occasionally (every 3 to 4 minutes).
- Remove from the heat. Stir in the sour cream.
- Serve immediately with fat-free grated Parmesan cheese on the side, if desired.

Yield: 12 (1-cup) servings

Calories: 225 (2% fat); Total Fat: 1 gm; Cholesterol: 3 mg; Carbohydrate: 45 gm; Dietary Fiber: 3 gm; Protein: 9 gm; Sodium: 438 mg
Diabetic Exchanges: 2 1/2 starch, 2 vegetable

Preparation time: 5 minutes or less
Cooking time: 25 minutes or less
Total time: 30 minutes or less

Menu Idea: For a vegetarian meal serve this with Creamy Blue Cheese Salad Dressing (page 64) from *Busy People's Down-Home Cooking Without the Down-Home Fat* on top of fresh tossed salad greens.

Italian Casserole Bake

I was in a real pinch. I was tired, overworked, and short on time and patience. When I got home everyone was hoping dinner was already done. Unfortunately, it was not! (I should have used one of my Busy People's Slow Cooker Cookbook *recipes that day.) I whipped this up in no time flat. By the time my daughter, Ashley, set the table, I had a happy family enjoying a tasty dinner.*

1 (12-ounce) bag Ground Meatless crumbles*	1 tablespoon dried Italian seasoning
1 (14-ounce) jar pizza sauce (I use Ragú)	Fat-free margarine spray
1 (10-ounce) can refrigerated pizza crust dough	1/2 cup (2 ounces) sliced fresh mushrooms
1/3 cup reduced-fat mozzarella cheese	Grated Parmesan cheese (optional)

- Preheat the oven to 400 degrees.
- Coat a 9 x 13-inch casserole dish with nonfat cooking spray.
- In the prepared dish, stir together the Ground Meatless and pizza sauce until well blended. Spread evenly on the bottom of the dish.
- Roll out the pizza dough on top of the pizza sauce mixture and stretch to cover the entire casserole.
- Sprinkle the mozzarella cheese evenly over the pizza dough.
- Sprinkle the Italian seasoning over the cheese and dough.
- Spray the top with about 15 sprays of the fat-free margarine.
- Arrange the mushroom slices over the top and bake on the top rack of the oven for 17 to 18 minutes or until the crust is golden brown.

- Let it sit for a couple of minutes before cutting into 6 servings.
- If desired, serve with Parmesan cheese on the side.

Note: I used hamburger-flavored veggie crumbles; however, for a much spicier dish use sausage-flavored crumbles. See page 16 for more information about Ground Meatless.

Yield: 6 servings

Calories: 241 (14% fat); Total Fat: 4 gm; Cholesterol: 3 mg; Carbohydrate: 32 gm;
Dietary Fiber: 5 gm; Protein: 19 gm; Sodium: 823 mg
Diabetic Exchanges: 2 starch, 1 vegetable, 2 very lean meat

Preparation time: 5 minutes or less
Cooking time: 18 minutes or less
Total time: 23 minutes or less

Menu Idea: I serve this with the Romaine and Pear Tossed Salad on page 146 of this book and the Italian Broccoli (page 74) from *Busy People's Down-Home Cooking Without the Down-Home Fat* for a meal the entire family can enjoy.

Italian Mini Meatloaves

These tasty little meatloaves are a cinch to make. They're one of my family's favorites.

1/2	teaspoon dried oregano	1	(14-ounce) jar light pizza sauce (I use Ragú Light)
1	pound ground eye of round		
2	egg whites	1/4	cup finely shredded Parmesan cheese (I use Kraft)
3/4	cup Italian breadcrumbs		
1/4	cup chopped fresh or frozen onion		

- Coat a nonstick skillet with nonfat cooking spray.
- In a bowl combine the oregano, ground eye of round, egg whites, breadcrumbs, and onion and stir until well mixed.
- Shape into six mini meatloaves and place in a skillet over medium heat.
- Cook, covered, for 10 minutes or until done, turning the meat over once.
- Pour the pizza sauce over each mini meatloaf and sprinkle with the cheese.
- Continue cooking for an additional 5 minutes.

Yield: 6 servings

Calories: 205 (24% fat); Total Fat: 5 gm; Cholesterol: 44 mg; Carbohydrate: 16 gm; Dietary Fiber: 2 gm; Protein: 23 gm; Sodium: 557 mg
Diabetic Exchanges: 2 1/2 lean meat, 1 starch

Preparation time: 5 minutes
Cooking time: 15 minutes
Total time: 20 minutes

Menu Idea: The Tomato Biscuits (page 59) from *Busy People's Low-Fat Cookbook* and Italian Zucchini on page 215 of this book are great with this Italian-inspired entrée!

Italian Burritos

Everyone is shocked that something this tasty and versatile can be made so quickly and with such simplicity.

1	(16-ounce) can fat-free refried beans	1	teaspoon dried Italian seasoning
2	ounces pepperoni, cut into tiny pieces	1/4	cup chopped frozen or fresh onion
2	(14-ounce) jars pizza sauce (I use Pizza Quick)	1	(8-ounce) package of fat-free mozzarella cheese
		20	(8-inch) fat-free tortillas

- In a medium bowl stir together the refried beans, pepperoni, pizza sauce, Italian seasoning, onion, and cheese until well mixed.
- Heat the tortillas in the microwave on high for 1 minute.
- Spoon 2 heaping tablespoons of the bean mixture into the center of each tortilla. Roll up the tortillas burrito-style and heat in the microwave for 15 seconds seam side down. If heating more than 1 burrito at a time, increase the time by 10 to 15 seconds per burrito.

Yield: 20 (1-burrito) servings

Calories: 196 (14% fat); Total Fat: 3 gm; Cholesterol: 4 mg; Carbohydrate: 31 gm;
Dietary Fiber: 4 gm; Protein: 10 gm; Sodium: 857 mg
Diabetic Exchanges: 2 starch, 1 very lean meat

Preparation time: 10 minutes or less
Cooking time: 5 minutes or less
Total time: 15 minutes or less

Menu Idea: Tomato Zing Salad (page 52) from *Busy People's Down-Home Cooking Without the Down-Home Fat* complements this easy meal nicely.

Chicken Mozzarella

It sounds hard to make, but actually it's quick, easy, and impressive.

4 ounces dry spaghetti or angel hair pasta	I (26-ounce) jar pasta sauce (I use Healthy Choice)
I pound skinless, boneless chicken breasts	$\frac{1}{4}$ cup shredded fat-free mozzarella cheese (I use Kraft)
$\frac{1}{2}$ cup Italian breadcrumbs	

- Preheat the oven to 450 degrees. Coat a baking sheet with nonfat cooking spray.
- Cook the pasta as directed on the package; drain.
- Pound the chicken to $\frac{1}{4}$ inch thick between sheets of wax paper. Rinse under running water.
- Coat the chicken with the breadcrumbs. Place on the prepared baking sheet and bake for 10 minutes.
- Microwave the pasta sauce for 3 minutes.
- Arrange the cooked pasta on a serving plate.
- Arrange the baked chicken on top of the pasta.
- Pour the pasta sauce over the chicken and pasta.
- Sprinkle with mozzarella cheese.
- If desired, cover with foil for a couple of minutes so that the heat from the hot pasta sauce and chicken melts the cheese.

Yield: 4 servings

Calories: 343 (6% fat); Total Fat: 2 gm; Cholesterol: 67 mg; Carbohydrate: 42 gm; Dietary Fiber: 4 gm; Protein: 36 gm; Sodium: 862 mg
Diabetic Exchanges: 3 very lean meat, 2 starch, 2 vegetable

Pork Mozzarella:

Make exactly the same as the Chicken Mozzarella recipe, but substitute 1 pound pork tenderloin steaks for the chicken breast.

Calories: 357 (13% fat); Total Fat: 5 gm; Cholesterol: 68 mg; Carbohydrate: 42 gm;
Dietary Fiber: 4 gm; Protein: 34 gm; Sodium: 836 mg
Diabetic Exchanges: 3 very lean meat, 2 starch, 2 vegetable

Preparation time: 10 minutes
Cooking time: 15 minutes
Total time: 25 minutes

Menu Ideas: Zucchini à la Parmesan (page 75) or Italian Broccoli (page 74) from *Busy People's Down-Home Cooking Without the Down-Home Fat* are great choices for this entrée.

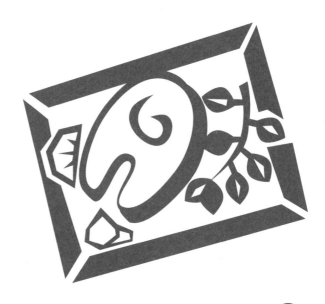

Chicken Parmesan with Vegetables

Usually Chicken Parmesan is served with pasta, but not in this filling and very satisfying Italian meal. You'll never miss the pasta or the added calories associated with pasta's carbohydrates. It's that satisfying.

1¹/₂ pounds chicken breast, cut into strips or 6 (4-ounce) chicken tenders	1 medium onion, thinly sliced and separated* (about 1 ¹/₂ cups)
1¹/₂ teaspoons dried oregano	1 (26-ounce) jar fat-free spaghetti sauce
1¹/₂ large red bell peppers, cut into thin strips (about 3 cups)*	1 tablespoon Splenda Granular
	¹/₄ cup shredded Parmesan cheese

- Pound the chicken to ¹/₂ inch thick between sheets of wax paper. (If you use the chicken tenders, also known as chicken strips, you can skip this step.)
- Place the chicken in a 12-inch nonstick skillet and sprinkle with the oregano.
- Cook the chicken, covered, over medium-high heat for 3 to 5 minutes. The chicken may get brown on the bottom.
- Turn over the chicken. Cover and continue cooking for 3 to 5 minutes or until the chicken is completely white on the inside of the thickest part of the chicken.
- Remove the chicken and place in a covered dish.
- Combine the bell pepper and onion in a dry skillet. Cover and cook over medium heat for 3 to 4 minutes, stirring occasionally. Some of the bell pepper will get brown and the onion will begin to caramelize and get brown as well. Moisture from the vegetables will steam them. No need for added water or fat.
- While the vegetables are cooking, set aside 1 cup of spaghetti sauce and save for another time. (A full jar is too much sauce.)
- Once the bell pepper is tender, but not soft, and the onion is cooked, reduce the heat to low.

- Pour the sauce over the vegetables.
- Sprinkle the Splenda over the sauce and vegetables. Stir and cook until well mixed and completely heated.
- Return the chicken to the skillet and stir to combine with the vegetables and sauce.
- Sprinkle with the cheese. Cover and cook until the cheese is completely melted, 1 to 2 minutes. Serve immediately.

Note: To save time, cut the red pepper and onion while the chicken is cooking. Other fresh vegetables such as sliced mushrooms and zucchini also taste great in this meal.

Yield: 6 servings (3 ounces cooked chicken and $\frac{1}{2}$ cup vegetables with sauce)

Calories: 191 (12% fat); Total Fat: 2 gm; Cholesterol: 68 mg; Carbohydrate: 12 gm; Dietary Fiber: 3 gm; Protein: 30 gm; Sodium: 397 mg
Diabetic Exchanges: 2$\frac{1}{2}$ vegetable, 3 very lean meat

Preparation time: 10 minutes or less
Cooking time: 20 minutes or less
Total time: 30 minutes or less

Menu Idea: This is a well-balanced meal as it is and nothing else is needed. However, for those who are not diabetic and want more carbohydrates the Italian Biscuits (page 28) along with the Portabello Garlic Mushrooms (page 13) both from *Busy People's Down-Home Cooking Without the Down-Home Fat* nicely complement this entrée.

Chicken Tacos

Marisela Delgado of San Antonio, Texas, says she converted a high-fat recipe her mother used to make. She started with fresh chicken. To save time I used canned.

¹/₂ large onion, chopped (about 1 cup)	¹/₂ cup chopped fresh cilantro
2 (12-ounce) cans chicken breast in water, undrained	1 (8-ounce, 12-count) package corn tortillas
2 tomatoes, chopped	2 cups shredded lettuce
	Taco sauce (optional)

- Coat a 12-inch nonstick pan with nonfat cooking spray.
- Cook the onion in the skillet, covered, over medium heat for 3 to 4 minutes, or until the onion is tender and translucent, stirring occasionally.
- Reduce the heat to medium low and add the chicken, tomatoes, and cilantro. Cook for 4 to 5 minutes or until all the ingredients are evenly cooked and the onion is tender.
- In a microwave, warm the corn tortillas for 5 to 7 seconds each.
- Fill each tortilla with ¹/₃ cup chicken mixture and fold.
- Top with shredded lettuce and taco sauce, if desired.

Yield: 12 servings (¹/₃ cup chicken taco mixture and 1 corn tortilla)

Calories: 109 (13% fat); Total Fat: 2 gm; Cholesterol: 24 mg; Carbohydrate: 11 gm; Dietary Fiber: 2 gm; Protein: 12 gm; Sodium: 255 mg
Diabetic Exchanges: ¹/₂ starch, 2 very lean meat

Preparation time: 10 minutes or less
Cooking time: 10 minutes or less
Total time: 20 minutes or less

Menu Ideas: I like serving an entire Mexican themed meal with this entrée. Try Taco Chowder (page 74) from *Busy People's Slow Cooker Cookbook.*

Mexicali Chicken

I converted this high-fat recipe sent in by Grace Du Prey of California into a quick, low-fat favorite.

1 pound skinless, boneless chicken breasts, all visible fat removed	1 (3-ounce) package fat-free cream cheese
1 (15-ounce) can beef chili (I use Healthy Choice)	1/4 cup mild thick and chunky salsa
	1 cup fat-free shredded Cheddar cheese (I use Healthy Choice)
	3 cups cooked hot rice

- In a 12-inch nonstick skillet, cook the chicken over medium-high heat for 3 to 4 minutes. Turn the chicken over and cook an additional 3 to 4 minutes or until cooked through.
- Remove the chicken from the heat. Cut into 1/4-inch-thick strips. Cut the strips into 1/2-inch-long pieces. Return the chicken to the skillet. Add the chili, cream cheese, and salsa and cook over medium-low heat, stirring constantly until the cream cheese is completely melted.
- Sprinkle with the Cheddar cheese. Cover and cook for 2 to 3 minutes. Serve over the cooked rice.

Note: To make into burritos, omit the rice and divide the mixture among 8 warmed fat-free tortillas.

Yield: 6 (1-burrito) servings

Calories: 209 (6% fat); Total Fat: 1 gm; Cholesterol: 38 mg; Carbohydrate: 24 gm; Dietary Fiber: 1 gm; Protein: 24 gm; Sodium: 331 mg
Diabetic Exchanges: 3 very lean meat, 1 1/2 starch
(as burritos) Calories: 252 (6% fat); Total Fat: 1 gm; Cholesterol: 38 mg; Carbohydrate: 32 gm; Dietary Fiber: 3 gm; Protein: 26 gm; Sodium: 670 mg
Diabetic Exchanges: 3 very lean meat, 2 starch

Preparation time: 10 minutes or less
Cooking time: 15 minutes or less (not including cooking the rice)
Total time: 25 minutes or less

Menu Idea: Start this festive meal off with a cup of hot Taco Vegetable Soup (page 62) from *Busy People's Slow Cooker Cookbook.*

Southwestern Angel Hair Pasta with Beef

The pasta-bilities of this entrée are endless! Try substituting your favorite types of small shaped pastas in place of the angel hair pasta.

1 pound ground eye of round	1 (8-ounce) can whole kernel corn, undrained
1 (14-ounce) can 98% fat-free beef broth	1 (15-ounce) can black beans, undrained
1 (16-ounce) jar thick and chunky salsa	1 (4.5-ounce) can chilies, undrained
1 (8-ounce) box angel hair pasta, broken into thirds	

- In a 12-inch nonstick skillet over high heat, cook the ground eye of round until fully cooked.
- Add the beef broth and salsa. Bring to a boil.
- Stir in the pasta. Reduce the heat to low. Cover and simmer for 8 to 10 minutes.
- Turn off the heat. Stir in the corn, black beans, chilies, and all the reserved liquids. Cover and let sit 2 minutes longer or until the corn and beans are thoroughly heated.
- Serve immediately.

Yield: 6 (1-cup) servings

Calories: 374 (21% fat); Total Fat: 9 gm; Cholesterol: 43 mg; Carbohydrate: 47 gm; Dietary Fiber: 6 gm; Protein: 24 gm; Sodium: 903 mg
Diabetic Exchanges: 3 starch, $2\frac{1}{2}$ lean meat

Southwestern Angel Hair Pasta with Chicken:
Substitute 1 pound chicken breast cut into bite-size pieces for the beef and substitute chicken broth for the beef broth.

Calories: 321 (5% fat); Total Fat: 2 gm; Cholesterol: 44 mg; Carbohydrate: 47 gm; Dietary Fiber: 6 gm; Protein: 27 gm; Sodium: 975 mg
Diabetic Exchanges: 3 starch, 2$\frac{1}{2}$ very lean meat

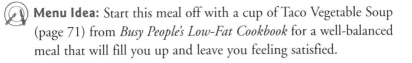

Preparation time: 5 minutes or less
Cooking time: 20 minutes or less
Total time: 25 minutes or less

Menu Idea: Start this meal off with a cup of Taco Vegetable Soup (page 71) from *Busy People's Low-Fat Cookbook* for a well-balanced meal that will fill you up and leave you feeling satisfied.

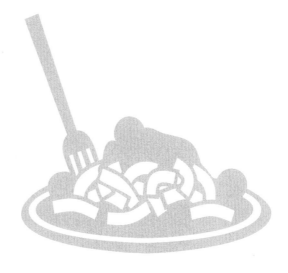

Southwestern Beef Gravy over Rice

This meal will stick to your bones but not your hips or thighs. Now isn't that a relief!

1 pound flank steak (also known as London broil)	1/4 cup mild chunky salsa
1 (15-ounce) can 98% fat-free chili	3 cups hot cooked brown rice
1/3 cup fat-free cream cheese	

- In a 12-inch nonstick skillet, cook the beef over medium-high heat for 3 to 4 minutes. Turn the steak over and cook for 3 to 4 minutes longer.
- Remove the steak from the heat and keep warm.
- In the skillet, combine the chili, cream cheese, and salsa and cook over medium-low heat. Stir frequently until the cream cheese is completely melted.
- Cut the steak against the grain into bite-size strips.
- Add the steak to the skillet, stirring until well mixed.
- Reduce the heat and cook, covered, over low heat for 2 to 3 minutes or until the meat is completely heated.
- Serve over the cooked rice.

Note: You can substitute a 12-ounce bag of frozen sausage-flavored Ground Meatless crumbles for the beef. (It is most likely too spicy for young children. I use Morningstar Farms brand found in the frozen meat section of the grocery store.)

Yield: 6 servings

(with steak) Calories: 299 (23% fat); Total Fat: 8 gm; Cholesterol: 49 mg; Carbohydrate: 31 gm; Dietary Fiber: 4 gm; Protein: 25 gm; Sodium: 521 mg Diabetic Exchanges: 2 starch, 3 lean meat
(with Ground Meatless) Calories: 275 (16% fat); Total Fat: 5 gm; Cholesterol: 11 mg; Carbohydrate: 36 gm; Dietary Fiber: 6 gm; Protein: 21 gm; Sodium: 847 mg Diabetic Exchanges: 2 1/2 starch, 2 very lean meat

Southwestern Beef Burritos:

Divide the mixture among twelve warmed fat-free flour tortillas. Omit the rice. Roll into burritos and serve with taco sauce on the side.

Yield: 12 (1-burrito) servings

(with steak) Calories: 215 (16% fat); Total Fat: 4 gm; Cholesterol: 24 mg; Carbohydrate: 28 gm; Dietary Fiber: 3 gm; Protein: 15 gm; Sodium: 598 mg
Diabetic Exchanges: 2 starch, 1$\frac{1}{2}$ lean meat

Preparation time: 5 minutes or less
Cooking time: 18 minutes or less
Total time: 23 minutes or less

Menu Idea: Serve with Crunchy Cucumbers with Cream (page 82) from *Busy People's Low-Fat Cookbook.* The coolness of this vegetable salad will complement the spicy flavor of the entrée.

Black Beans & Rice

It's a southern dish made in a fraction of the original time.

2 teaspoons minced garlic (I use the kind in a jar)	1/2 cup chopped frozen or fresh onion
1 teaspoon liquid smoke (found with barbecue sauce)	1 (15-ounce) can black beans, undrained (I use Progresso)
4 ounces extra lean cooked ham, cut into tiny pieces (lunch meat is fine)	1 cup instant long grain white rice

- Combine the garlic, liquid smoke, ham, onion, and black beans with liquid in a 4½-quart saucepan over medium-high heat. Bring to a full boil.
- Stir in the rice, cover, and remove from the heat.
- Let it sit for 5 minutes. Serve hot.

Yield: 4 (1-cup) servings

Calories: 225 (14% fat); Total Fat: 4 gm; Cholesterol: 13 mg; Carbohydrate: 34 gm; Dietary Fiber: 6 gm; Protein: 13 gm; Sodium: 736 mg
Diabetic Exchanges: 1½ very lean meat, 2½ starch

Yield: 8 (½-cup) servings

Calories: 112 (14% fat); Total Fat: 2 gm; Cholesterol: 7 mg; Carbohydrate: 17 gm; Dietary Fiber: 3 gm; Protein: 7 gm; Sodium: 368 mg
Diabetic Exchanges: ½ very lean meat, 1 starch

Preparation time: 10 minutes or less
Cooking time: 10 minutes or less
Total time: 20 minutes or less

Menu Idea: For a fine southern-style meal serve this with Southwestern Corn Bread (page 40) from *Busy People's Slow Cooker Cookbook* (yes, it's baked in a slow cooker!) and Tomato Zing Salad (page 52) from *Busy People's Down-Home Cooking Without the Down-Home Fat.*

Open-Faced Warm Chicken Salad Sandwiches

This recipe was sent in by Angie Avers of Maumee, Ohio, with a few changes of my own. I give her full credit for this delicious and easy recipe.

1 (8-ounce) can water chestnuts, drained and finely chopped	3 tablespoons fat-free creamy salad dressing (I use Miracle Whip Free)
1 (10-ounce) can chunk chicken breast, in water	1 tablespoon honey mustard (I use Grey Poupon)
1/2 cup finely chopped broccoli (fresh or frozen)	2 (7.5-ounce) cans refrigerated Pillsbury biscuits
1/3 cup shredded fat-free mozzarella cheese (I use Kraft)	

- Preheat the oven to 350 degrees. Coat a baking sheet with nonfat cooking spray.
- In a mixing bowl combine the water chestnuts, chicken, broccoli, cheese, salad dressing, and honey mustard until well mixed.
- Flatten thirteen biscuits to the size of your palm. (If desired, save the remaining seven biscuits for future use.)
- Lay the flattened biscuits on the prepared baking sheet.
- Top each with the chicken mixture.
- Bake for 15 minutes.

Yield: 6½ servings (2 sandwiches per serving)

Calories: 182 (13% fat); Total Fat: 3 gm; Cholesterol: 19 mg; Carbohydrate: 25 gm; Dietary Fiber: 2 gm; Protein: 13 gm; Sodium: 652 mg
Diabetic Exchanges: 1 very lean meat, 1½ starch, 1 vegetable

Preparation time: 10 minutes or less
Cooking time: 15 minutes
Total time: 25 minutes or less

Menu Idea: The Polynesian Fruit Salad (page 78) from *Busy People's Low-Fat Cookbook* and a Fresh Broccoli Salad (page 53) from *Busy People's Down-Home Cooking Without the Down-Home Fat* will make these sandwiches into a complete meal everyone will love.

Chicken-Fried Steak

I don't know why it's called chicken-fried steak. It's made of beef. I bake it until it's crispy. It is so good!

1/3	cup all-purpose flour	2	tablespoons skim milk
1	teaspoon Lawry's seasoned salt	6	(1/4-inch) eye of round steaks
3/4	cup seasoned breadcrumbs		(about 1 pound)
2	egg whites, beaten	1	(12-ounce) jar fat-free chicken gravy (optional)

- Preheat the oven to 400 degrees. Coat a baking sheet with nonfat cooking spray.
- In a bowl stir together the flour, seasoned salt, and breadcrumbs.
- In a separate bowl beat together the egg whites and milk.
- Coat the meat in the breadcrumb mixture and dip into the egg mixture. Then re-dip into the breadcrumb mixture.
- Place the breaded meat on the prepared baking sheet. Spray the top of the meat with nonfat cooking spray.
- Bake for 10 minutes. Turn over. Spray the top of the meat with nonfat cooking spray. Bake an additional 10 minutes. Breading will be crispy and slightly golden brown when done.
- Microwave the gravy for 2 minutes or until fully heated. Pour 1/4 cup gravy over each steak before serving.

Yield: 6 servings

Calories: 174 (19% fat); Total Fat: 4 gm; Cholesterol: 46 mg; Carbohydrate: 14 gm; Dietary Fiber: 1 gm; Protein: 20 gm; Sodium: 804 mg
Diabetic Exchanges: 2 very lean meat, 1 starch

Preparation time: 7 minutes or less
Cooking time: 23 minutes or less
Total time: 30 minutes or less

Menu Idea: *Busy People's Down-Home Cooking Without the Down-Home Fat* has home-style side dishes such as Potatoes à la Larry (easy mashed potatoes) on page 77 and Mama's Green Beans on page 71 that'll accompany this entrée perfectly!

Oriental Vegetables & Rice

Don't confuse this with fried rice. This has its own unique flavor. The little bit of sesame oil I use will give this delicious dish just a little bit of fat, but a lot of good flavor.

2	cups fat-free, reduced-sodium chicken broth	4	ounces extra-lean thinly sliced ham, cut into 1/2-inch squares
1	pound frozen stir-fry vegetables (I use Flav-R-Pac)	2	cups instant white long-grain rice (I use Minute)
1	teaspoon sesame oil		Light soy sauce for seasoning (optional)

- In a 3-quart saucepan over high heat, bring the chicken broth, vegetables, and sesame oil to a full boil.
- Remove from the heat. Stir in the ham and rice.
- Cover and let sit for 5 minutes.
- If desired, serve with light soy sauce on the side.

Note: You can substitute 3/4 pound cooked chicken for the ham.

Yield: 4 (1 1/2-cup) servings

(with ham) Calories: 300 (10% fat); Total Fat: 3 gm; Cholesterol: 13 mg; Carbohydrate: 52 gm; Dietary Fiber: 5 gm; Protein: 14 gm; Sodium: 688 mg
Diabetic Exchanges: 1 very lean meat, 2 1/2 starch, 3 vegetable
(with chicken) Calories: 403 (11% fat); Total Fat: 5 gm; Cholesterol: 72 mg; Carbohydrate: 52 gm; Dietary Fiber: 5 gm; Protein: 35 gm; Sodium: 346 mg
Diabetic Exchanges: 3 very lean meat, 2 1/2 starch, 3 vegetable

Preparation time: 10 minutes or less
Cooking time: 14 minutes or less
Total time: 24 minutes or less

Menu Idea: This is a complete meal in itself. For a light dessert serve Melon Salad on page 138 of this book.

Stuffed Harvest Acorn Squash

Beautiful to see and comforting to eat, these squash can be prepared days in advance. Refrigerate and cook individually in the microwave for about five minutes per acorn half when needed.

3	acorn squash, cut in half vertically and seeded	1/4	cup light maple syrup
1	(6-ounce) box pork-flavored stuffing (I use Stove Top)	1	pound fat-free ham, cut into 1/4-inch pieces
2	cups hot water	1	large apple, unpeeled and cut into 1/4-inch pieces (any apple except Red Delicious)
2	tablespoons butter-flavored sprinkles, dry		

Microwave method:

- Arrange the acorn squash on a microwave-safe plate. Set aside.
- In a large bowl, combine the stuffing with the seasoning packet, water, and butter-flavored sprinkles until well mixed.
- Stir in the maple syrup, ham, and apple until well mixed.
- Fill each squash half with the prepared stuffing.
- Spray the tops of squash and stuffing with nonfat cooking spray, to prevent waxed paper from sticking and to help prevent drying.
- Cover each stuffed squash with wax paper.
- Cook on high in a carousel microwave for 5 to 7 minutes per squash.
- The squash will be soft (yet slightly firm) to the touch when ready to eat. If more cooking time is needed simply cook 1 minute longer per squash half.

Oven method:

- It will take a lot longer, but if you would prefer to cook the squash in the oven, follow the recipe exactly. Cover the top of the squash half with aluminum foil. Place the squash in a glass baking dish that has $\frac{1}{2}$ cup of water in the bottom of it. Bake at 350 degrees for 1 hour.

Slow cooker method:

- Wrap each squash half in aluminum foil and place in a slow cooker. Add 1 cup of water in the slow cooker. Cook, covered, on high for 4 hours or on low for 8 to 9 hours.

Yield: 6 stuffed acorn squash halves

Calories: 296 (4% fat); Total Fat: 1 gm; Cholesterol: 24 mg; Carbohydrate: 56 gm; Dietary Fiber: 5 gm; Protein: 17 gm; Sodium: 1484 mg
Diabetic Exchanges: 2 very lean meat, 3 starch, $\frac{1}{2}$ fruit

Preparation time: 9 minutes or less
Cooking time: (microwave method): 21 minutes or less
Total time: 30 minutes or less

Menu Idea: The Red Wine Vinaigrette Cucumber Salad (page 49) from *Busy People's Down-Home Cooking Without the Down-Home Fat* tastes terrific with this recipe.

Cornmeal & Ranch Flavored Chicken Strips

If you don't want the expense and high fat of store-bought, prepackaged chicken strips, then you may want to give this quick little recipe a try. You'll save oodles of money and it will only take about four or five more minutes to prepare than prepackaged brands.

½ cup self-rising cornmeal mix 1 envelope ranch salad dressing mix (do not make as directed)	2 pounds skinless, boneless chicken strips (also called tenders)—not frozen Ketchup, mustard, or barbeque sauce for dipping (optional)

- Preheat the oven to 400 degrees.
- Line an 11 x 17-inch jelly roll pan with aluminum foil. Coat the foil with nonfat cooking spray.
- Stir the cornmeal and ranch salad dressing mix together in a medium bowl until well mixed.
- Lightly coat the chicken with the cornmeal breading one piece at a time. The chicken strips will be moist, which will hold the seasoning onto the chicken.
- Place the prepared chicken strips on the pan. Spray the chicken strips with nonfat cooking spray.
- Bake on the top rack of the oven for 10 minutes.
- Turn the chicken strips over. Coat the tops of the chicken with nonfat cooking spray.
- Bake another 3 to 5 minutes or until the chicken is completely white in the thickest part.
- Serve with ketchup, mustard, or barbeque sauce for dipping.

Yield: 8 (3-ounce cooked) servings

Calories: 171 (10% fat); Total Fat: 2 gm; Cholesterol: 66 mg; Carbohydrate: 10 gm; Dietary Fiber: 1 gm; Protein: 27 gm; Sodium: 641 mg
Diabetic Exchanges: $\frac{1}{2}$ starch, 3 very lean meat

Preparation time: 10 minutes or less
Cooking time: 15 minutes or less
Total time: 25 minutes or less

Menu Idea: This easy finger-food entrée is a hit, especially with children. To help with cleanup, I make this entire meal a finger-food dinner by serving with fresh veggie sticks and my Buttermilk Ranch Salad Dressing (page 53) from *Busy People's Low-Fat Cookbook* for dipping.

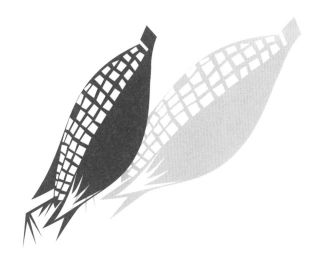

Pork Hash

This is a terrific way to use leftover cooked pork tenderloin. One taste of this and you may never want to eat unhealthy, higher calorie corned beef hash again.

1 **pound frozen fat-free hash browns**	**Ground black pepper**
1 **pound cooked pork tenderloin, shredded**	

- Coat a 12-inch nonstick skillet with nonfat cooking spray.
- Cook the hash browns in the skillet over medium-high heat. With the back of a spatula press down on the hash browns and then cover to cook more quickly. Stir occasionally to prevent burning.
- Add the pork and cook until heated through.
- Stir in the pepper to taste until well mixed.
- Serve immediately.

Yield: 4 (8-ounce) servings

Calories: 273 (18% fat); Total Fat: 6 gm; Cholesterol: 90 mg; Carbohydrate: 20 gm; Dietary Fiber: 2 gm; Protein: 34 gm; Sodium: 88 mg
Diabetic Exchanges: $1\frac{1}{2}$ starch, 4 very lean meat

Preparation time: 5 minutes or less
Cooking time: 20 minutes or less
Total time: 25 minutes or less

Menu Idea: The Melon Salad on page 138 of this book along with the Mint Tea (page 208) from *Busy People's Down-Home Cooking Without the Down-Home Fat* make this a great meal any time of day.

Garlic Beef

The wonderful aroma calls everyone to the table before it's even time to eat.

I	teaspoon sesame oil	I	tablespoon minced garlic (I use the kind in a jar)
I	pound eye of round, cut into thin strips	2	tablespoons light soy sauce
I	(10-ounce) package frozen chopped broccoli	¼	teaspoon ground black pepper

- In a 12-inch nonstick skillet, heat the sesame oil over high heat. Add the eye of round, broccoli, garlic, soy sauce, and pepper and cook until the beef is fully cooked, 18 to 20 minutes.
- Serve hot.

Yield: 4 servings

Calories: 189 (30% fat); Total Fat: 6 gm; Cholesterol: 61 mg; Carbohydrate: 5 gm; Dietary Fiber: 2 gm; Protein: 28 gm; Sodium: 330 mg
Diabetic Exchanges: 3 lean meat, 1 vegetable

Preparation time: 5 minutes or less
Cooking time: 20 minutes or less
Total time: 25 minutes or less

Menu Idea: This is good served over rice with the Spinach Orange Salad on page 141 in this book on the side.

Chicken with Cool & Creamy Lime Sauce

Don't be surprised if this becomes one of those favorite quickie meals you'll want to make again and again. It is very versatile.

2 limes, divided	1/2 cup fat-free sour cream
I pound skinless, boneless chicken breasts, cut into 1/4-inch-wide strips about 2 inches long	I tablespoon ranch salad dressing mix, dry

- With your hand, roll the limes firmly on the countertop to soften and release their juices.
- Cut the limes in half and squeeze the juice of 1 lime into a 12-inch nonstick skillet over medium-high heat.
- Add the chicken and cook until white, 3 to 7 minutes. Cover the skillet to help the chicken cook more quickly.
- While the chicken is cooking, in a small bowl mix together the juice of the remaining lime, sour cream, and ranch dressing mix.
- Once the chicken is fully cooked, remove from the skillet. Spoon 2 tablespoons of the prepared lime cream over each serving.

Yield: 4 servings (3 ounces cooked chicken and 2 tablespoons lime sauce)

Calories: 171 (8% fat); Total Fat: 1 gm; Cholesterol: 71 mg; Carbohydrate: 9 gm; Dietary Fiber: 0 gm; Protein: 28 gm; Sodium: 375 mg
Diabetic Exchanges: 1/2 other carbohydrate, 3 very lean meat

Preparation time: 5 minutes or less
Cooking time: 7 minutes or less
Total time: 12 minutes or less

Menu Ideas: I like to serve this with fat-free flour tortillas, shredded lettuce, and chopped fresh tomatoes so everyone can make their own lime chicken roll-ups. However, some people like it served over a bed of lettuce as a salad fit for a meal. Whatever way you choose, I'm sure you'll like it.

Lemon-Herb Chicken Cutlets

The zip from the lemon gives the herbs an extra kick!

8 (4-ounce) chicken breasts*	$\frac{1}{2}$ teaspoon dried thyme
1 teaspoon lemon pepper seasoning	$\frac{1}{2}$ teaspoon dried basil
	$\frac{1}{2}$ teaspoon dried parsley

- Pound the chicken breasts between two pieces of wax paper until they are $\frac{1}{2}$ inch thick.
- Combine the lemon pepper, thyme, basil, and parsley in a large zip-top plastic bag and shake until well mixed.
- Lightly sprinkle both sides of each chicken cutlet with the seasoning blend.
- Grill or broil the chicken at medium-high heat for 3 to 4 minutes on each side. The chicken will be white and juicy on the inside when fully cooked.

Note: If your chicken breasts are too thick and weigh more than 4 ounces each: Press your hand down on top of the chicken breast and cut the breast horizontally in half with a very sharp knife.

Yield: 8 (3-ounce cooked) servings

Calories: 125 (11% fat); Total Fat: 1 gm; Cholesterol: 66 mg; Carbohydrate: 0 gm; Dietary Fiber: 0 gm; Protein: 26 gm; Sodium: 114 mg
Diabetic Exchanges: 3 very lean meat

Preparation time: 10 minutes or less
Cooking time: 8 minutes or less
Total time: 18 minutes or less

Menu Idea: For a fantastic meal you can put together in a jiffy that'll have your guests "oooing" and "ahhing" (and thinking you've been slaving in the kitchen all day) serve this with the World's Easiest Spinach Salad on page 142 along with the White Chocolate Mousse on page 272 both from this cookbook and the Creamed Green Beans with Ham (page 111) from *Busy People's Low-Fat Cookbook.*

Herb Chicken (or Turkey) Cutlets

Chicken cutlets are a fancy term used to describe chicken breasts that have been cut up. If you are unable to find small chicken breasts then slice a thick chicken breast in half.

8 (4-ounce) skinless, boneless chicken (or turkey) breasts	1/2 teaspoon dried basil
1/2 teaspoon dried thyme	1/4 teaspoon ground black pepper
1/2 teaspoon dried rosemary	1/4 teaspoon garlic salt

- Pound the chicken breasts between two pieces of wax paper until they are 1/2 inch thick.
- Combine the thyme, rosemary, basil, black pepper, and garlic salt in a large zip-top plastic bag and shake until well mixed.
- Lightly sprinkle both sides of each chicken cutlet with the herb blend.
- Grill or broil the chicken at medium-high heat for 3 to 4 minutes on each side. The chicken will be white and juicy on the inside when fully cooked.

Yield: 8 (3-ounce cooked) servings

(with chicken) Calories: 126 (11% fat); Total Fat: 1 gm; Cholesterol: 66 mg; Carbohydrate: 0 gm; Dietary Fiber: 0 gm; Protein: 26 gm; Sodium: 104 mg
Diabetic Exchanges: 3 very lean meat
(with turkey) Calories: 126 (8% fat); Total Fat: 1 gm; Cholesterol: 77 mg; Carbohydrate: 0 gm; Dietary Fiber: 0 gm; Protein: 27 gm; Sodium: 80 mg
Diabetic Exchanges: 3 very lean meat

Preparation time: 10 minutes or less
Cooking time: 8 minutes or less
Total time: 18 minutes or less

Menu Idea: This is one of those wonderful entrées that is low in fat and calories and allows room for higher calorie side dishes such as the Sweet and Sour Fresh Vegetable Garden Salad (page 83) and Peppered Potato Salad (page 105) both from *Busy People's Low-Fat Cookbook.*

Italian Zucchini

Here's a delicious way to use some of that zucchini from your garden to make a meatless main dish.

4 cups sliced zucchini	1 medium onion, chopped, or 1 cup
1 (26-ounce) jar spaghetti sauce	frozen chopped onion
1 (12-ounce) bag sausage-flavored Ground Meatless*	

- Preheat a slow cooker on high and spray with nonfat cooking spray.
- Combine the zucchini, spaghetti sauce, sausage crumbles, and onion in the slow cooker.
- Cover and cook on high for 4 hours.

*Note: See page 16 for more information on Ground Meatless

Yield: 8 (1-cup) servings

Calories: 137 (23% fat); Total Fat: 4 gm; Cholesterol: 0 mg; Carbohydrate: 16 gm; Dietary Fiber: 4 gm; Protein: 11 gm; Sodium: 703 mg
Diabetic Exchanges: 1 starch, 1 lean meat

Preparation time: 10 minutes

Menu Ideas: This can be served as a meatless spaghetti sauce over cooked pasta or eaten plain. I like Garlic Toast (page 61) from *Busy People's Low-Fat Cookbook* with this Italian entrée, and a tossed salad with fat-free Italian salad dressing.

Turkey Cutlets with Zesty Cranberry Sauce

The ingredients will surprise you. The flavor will delight you!

4 (4-ounce) turkey cutlets	2 teaspoons horseradish
1/4 cup whole cranberry sauce	

- Cook the turkey cutlets, covered, in a 12-inch nonstick skillet for 3 to 5 minutes over medium-high heat.
- Stir the cranberry sauce and horseradish together until well blended.
- Turn over the turkey cutlets. Spread 1 tablespoon of the cranberry-horseradish sauce over each turkey cutlet.
- Reduce the heat to medium. Continue cooking, covered, for another 3 to 5 minutes or until the turkey is white and juicy in the center.
- Serve immediately.

Yield: 4 servings (3-ounces cooked cutlets and 1 tablespoon sauce)

Calories: 152 (7% fat); Total Fat: 1 gm; Cholesterol: 77 mg; Carbohydrate: 7 gm; Dietary Fiber: 0 gm; Protein: 27 gm; Sodium: 62 mg
Diabetic Exchanges: 1/2 other carbohydrate, 3 very lean meat

Preparation time: 5 minutes or less
Cooking time: 10 minutes or less
Total time: 15 minutes or less

Menu Idea: The cool and refreshing taste of the Creamy Cucumbers (page 50) from *Busy People's Down-Home Cooking Without the Down-Home Fat* along with the Garlic Red Skins (page 117) from *Busy People's Low-Fat Cookbook* are nice complements to this entrée.

Kielbasa & Rice

Sauerkraut lovers will love this dish.

1 (14-ounce) package fat-free Polish kielbasa, cut into tiny pieces (I use Butterball)	1 (14.5-ounce) can no-salt-added stewed tomatoes, cut into bite-size pieces*
1 (16-ounce) can sauerkraut, rinsed and squeezed dry	2 1/2 cups low-sodium vegetable juice cocktail (I use V-8)
	2 cups instant rice

- In a 3-quart nonstick pan, bring the kielbasa, sauerkraut, tomatoes, and vegetable juice to a full boil, stirring occasionally.
- Stir in the rice and cover.
- Remove from the heat and let sit for 5 minutes.

Note: The easiest, quickest way to cut tomatoes is to leave them in the can. Insert a knife in the opened can and cut.

Yield: 5 servings

Calories: 283 (0% fat); Total Fat: 0 gm; Cholesterol: 34 mg; Carbohydrate: 53 gm; Dietary Fiber: 2 gm; Protein: 17 gm; Sodium: 1423 mg
Diabetic Exchanges: 2 very lean meat, 2 1/2 starch, 3 vegetable

Preparation time: 5 minutes or less
Cooking time: 18 minutes or less
Total time: 23 minutes or less

Menu Idea: A meal in itself; however, if you'd like a dessert a serving of Melon Salad on page 138 of this book will work just fine.

Bacon, Mushroom & Onion Gravy

You probably are thinking this just sounds way too fattening to be able to eat on a diabetic diet or weight loss program. Although it tastes like it, the wonderful news is that it's not.

3 cups cold skim milk	1/2 cup reduced-fat real bacon bits (from a jar)
3 tablespoons cornstarch	
3 tablespoons imitation butter-flavored sprinkles, dry	3 1/2 cups sliced fresh mushrooms
1/2 cup finely chopped onion (fresh or frozen)	1/2 cup shredded Parmesan cheese

- In a 12-inch nonstick skillet over medium heat, briskly whisk the milk, cornstarch, and butter sprinkles together until everything is completely dissolved.
- Stir in the onion and bacon. Cook for 5 to 10 minutes, stirring frequently to prevent lumps. The sauce will thicken as it cooks. The longer it cooks the thicker it will become. Be patient. You can't rush this process.
- When thickened, stir in the mushrooms. Cover and continue to cook, stirring frequently but not constantly, for another 5 to 10 minutes or until the mushroom slices are tender. The thinner the mushrooms are sliced the quicker they will become tender.
- Stir in the cheese. Keep cooking, stirring continuously, until the cheese is thoroughly melted.
- Serve immediately.

Note: If desired season with light salt or Mrs. Dash salt-free seasoning and pepper.

Yield: 6 (1-cup) servings

Calories: 149 (26% fat); Total Fat: 4 gm; Cholesterol: 14 mg; Carbohydrate: 16 gm;
Dietary Fiber: 1 gm; Protein: 12 gm; Sodium: 693 mg
Diabetic Exchanges: $^1\!/_2$ starch, $^1\!/_2$ skim milk, 1 lean meat

Preparation time: 5 minutes or less
Cooking time: 22 minutes or less
Total time: 27 minutes or less

Menu Idea: For each serving I like to serve 1 cup of this over $^1\!/_2$ cup of my homemade Mashed Potatoes Deluxe (page 119) from *Busy People's Low-Fat Cookbook* along with my Orange Cranberry Jell-O Salad (page 46) from *Busy People's Down-Home Cooking Without the Down-Home Fat* and a fresh tossed salad.

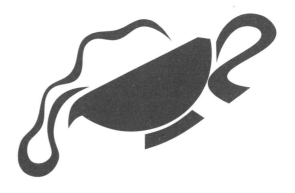

Simple Chicken Strips

These lightly breaded chicken strips are super-easy and simple to prepare!

3/4 cup crushed Special K cereal

1/4 cup reduced-fat baking mix (I use Bisquick)

1 teaspoon Mrs. Dash salt-free seasoning

1 pound skinless, boneless chicken tenders or strips about 1/2 inch wide and 2 to 3 inches long

- Preheat the oven to 400 degrees.
- Line a jelly roll pan with aluminum foil. Spray the foil with nonfat cooking spray.
- In a medium bowl stir together the cereal, baking mix, and seasoning.
- Rinse the chicken with water. Dip the chicken pieces into the cereal mixture, coating the chicken strips lightly. The dampness of the wet chicken is what will make the seasoning stick to the chicken.
- Place the coated chicken strips onto the prepared baking sheet, making sure the edges do not touch each other. Spray the tops of the chicken lightly with nonfat cooking spray. Bake for 8 to 10 minutes.
- Turn the strips and spray again lightly with nonfat cooking spray.
- Bake an additional 2 to 3 minutes or until the center is white.

Yield: 4 (3-ounce cooked) servings

Calories: 175 (11% fat); Total Fat: 2 gm; Cholesterol: 66 mg; Carbohydrate: 9 gm; Dietary Fiber: 0 gm; Protein: 28 gm; Sodium: 203 mg
Diabetic Exchanges: 1/2 starch, 3 very lean meat

Preparation time: 10 minutes or less
Cooking time: 13 minutes or less
Total time: 23 minutes or less

Menu Idea: Crunchy Cucumbers with Cream (page 82) and Peppered Potato Salad (page 105) both from *Busy People's Low-Fat Cookbook* make a good meal for either lunch or dinner. These are also a big hit at parties where only appetizers are served.

Sausage & Potato Skillet Dinner

Meat and potato lovers will never know this is a vegetarian dish. It tastes that good.

1/2 cup chopped red onion	1 (12-ounce) bag sausage-flavored Ground Meatless crumbles (I use Morningstar Farms)
2 tablespoons reduced-fat butter	
1 pound precooked, frozen, fat-free hash browns	1 (15-ounce) can whole kernel corn, drained

- In a large nonstick skillet, cook the onion in the butter over medium-high heat for about 2 minutes or until tender.
- Add the hash browns. Stir until well mixed. Press the potatoes and onion mixture firmly with the back of a spatula. Cook for about 5 to 6 minutes. Turn the potatoes over. Stir and continue cooking until golden brown.
- Stir in the sausage crumbles and corn. Continue cooking for 3 to 4 minutes or until fully heated.

Note: Ground Meatless is a vegetarian product that tastes like cooked, crumbled hamburger. It does not need to be cooked before adding to the recipe. See page 16 for more information. You can substitute low-fat turkey Italian sausage for the Ground Meatless if desired.

Yield: 5 (1-cup) servings

<u>(with Ground Meatless)</u> Calories: 276 (21% fat); Total Fat: 7 gm; Cholesterol: 8 mg; Carbohydrate: 39 gm; Dietary Fiber: 6 gm; Protein: 18 gm; Sodium: 688 mg
Diabetic Exchanges: 2$\frac{1}{2}$ starch, 2 lean meat
<u>(with low-fat turkey Italian sausage)</u> Calories: 273 (31 % fat); Total Fat: 10 gm; Cholesterol: 65 mg; Carbohydrate: 33 gm; Dietary Fiber: 3 gm; Protein: 14 gm; Sodium: 714 mg
Diabetic Exchanges: 2 starch, 2 lean meat, $\frac{1}{2}$ fat

Preparation time: 5 minutes or less
Cooking time: 10 minutes or less
Total time: 15 minutes or less

Menu Idea: For a great meal, serve this with the Mushrooms and Asparagus on page 129 of *Busy People's Low-Fat Cookbook.*

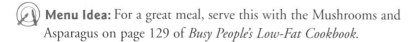

Cheeseburger Slow Cooker Casserole

This is a very good meatless dish. No one will guess there's not any meat in it. I took an original high-fat, meat-based entrée and converted it to this yummy low-fat, vegetarian entrée, which is every bit as good as the conventional recipe but with a lot fewer calories.

1 cup chopped onion (fresh or frozen)	1/2 cup reduced-fat baking mix (I use Bisquick)
1 (12-ounce) bag Ground Meatless veggie crumbles* (I use Morningstar Farms)	1 cup skim milk
1 cup shredded fat-free Cheddar cheese	1/2 cup liquid egg substitute (I use Egg Beaters) or 4 egg whites

- Preheat the slow cooker on high and coat with nonfat cooking spray.
- Cook the onion in the microwave for 2 minutes. (Add 30 seconds if using frozen onions.)
- Combine the cooked onions with the Ground Meatless and spread in the bottom of the slow cooker.
- Sprinkle the cheese on top.
- In a medium mixing bowl stir together the baking mix, milk, and egg substitute or egg whites until well blended.
- Pour the mixture over the ingredients in the slow cooker. Cover and cook on high for 2½ hours or until a knife inserted in the center comes out clean.

Note: My family really likes this recipe as is, but 1 pound ground round can be substituted for Ground Meatless. (See page 16.) If ground round is used it must be browned and well drained before adding to the recipe. The onion can be browned with the meat.

Yield: 4 (1-cup) servings

<u>(with Ground Meatless)</u> Calories: 258 (4% fat); Total Fat: 1 gm; Cholesterol: 6 mg; Carbohydrate: 27 gm; Dietary Fiber: 5 gm; Protein: 34 gm; Sodium: 768 mg
Diabetic Exchanges: $1\frac{1}{2}$ starch, 1 vegetable, 4 very lean meat
<u>(with ground round)</u> Calories: 255 (15% fat); Total Fat: 4 gm; Cholesterol: 50 mg; Carbohydrate: 19 gm; Dietary Fiber: 1 gm; Protein: 34 gm; Sodium: 574 mg
Diabetic Exchanges: 1 starch, 1 vegetable, 4 very lean meat

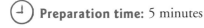 **Preparation time:** 5 minutes

Menu Idea: To complete this meal the Crunchy Cucumbers with Cream (page 82) and the Bacon, Lettuce & Tomato Salad (page 96) both from *Busy People's Low-Fat Cookbook* taste really good with this.

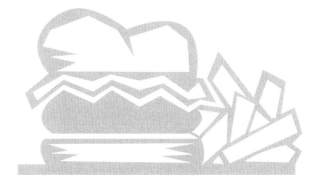

Heartland Casserole

This is a basic heartland casserole that's made quickly and easily.

1 (8-ounce) package pasta shells	8 ounces Ground Meatless* crumbles (I use Morningstar Farms)
1 (4-ounce) can mushroom stems and pieces, undrained	
1 (14.5-ounce) can no-salt-added diced tomatoes, undrained	1/2 cup chopped frozen green bell pepper (optional)
1 (15-ounce) can reduced-fat cream of mushroom soup (not the condensed kind)	1/2 cup chopped onion (optional)
	4 slices fat-free sharp Cheddar singles, quartered (I use Kraft Free)

- In a 2½-quart or larger microwave-safe casserole dish, mix together the pasta shells, mushrooms, tomatoes, soup, and Ground Meatless.
- Add the green bell pepper and onion if using. Add 1 cup hot water.
- Cook, covered, in a carousel microwave on high for 10 minutes, stirring once after 5 minutes.
- Stir in the cheese until well mixed. Continue cooking on high, covered, for an additional 5 minutes.
- Stir, cover, and let sit for 3 to 5 minutes.

*Note: If you would prefer, you can use cooked ground eye of round. See page 16 for more information on Ground Meatless.

Yield: 4 servings

(with Ground Meatless) Calories: 250 (4% fat); Total Fat: 1 gm; Cholesterol: 2 mg; Carbohydrate: 42 gm; Dietary Fiber: 3 gm; Protein: 17 gm; Sodium: 581 mg
Diabetic Exchanges: 2 very lean meat, 2 starch, 2 vegetable
(with eye of round) Calories: 257 (9% fat); Total Fat: 3 gm; Cholesterol: 22 mg; Carbohydrate: 39 gm; Dietary Fiber: 2 gm; Protein: 19 gm; Sodium: 421 mg
Diabetic Exchanges (same for all variations): 2 very lean meat, 2 starch, 2 vegetable

Preparation time: 10 minutes or less
Cooking time: 15 minutes or less
Total time: 25 minutes or less

Menu Idea: I like the Crunchy Cucumbers with Cream (page 82) from *Busy People's Low-Fat Cookbook* with this casserole.

Lazy Unstuffed Cabbage

Here's another delicious meatless main dish that no one will ever know is vegetarian.

1 (12-ounce) bag Ground Meatless crumbles	2 cups shredded cabbage, or about 8 ounces prepackaged shredded coleslaw mix
2 teaspoons dried onion flakes	1 cup instant rice*
	2 cups tomato juice

- Coat a slow cooker with nonfat cooking spray.
- Stir together the meatless crumbles, onion flakes, cabbage, rice, and tomato juice until well mixed.
- Cook on high for 3 hours.

*Note: If using regular rice, cook for 1 hour longer. The flavor is very good! See note on page 16 for more information on Ground Meatless.

Yield: 6 (1-cup) servings

Calories: 150 (0% fat); Total Fat: 0 gm; Cholesterol: 0mg; Carbohydrate: 22 gm; Dietary Fiber: 4 gm; Protein: 14 gm; Sodium: 492 mg
Diabetic Exchanges: 1 starch, 1$\frac{1}{2}$ vegetable, 1 very lean meat

Preparation time: 5 minutes

Menu Idea: This is a complete meal in itself and is a good source of both lean protein and carbohydrates. However, if you want something more with your meal try the fresh Melon Salad on page 138 of this book.

Barbequed Pork & Potato Skillet Casserole

This is for the meat and potato lover who loves barbeque. For fun, serve on pie pans instead of plates with gingham handkerchiefs as napkins and coffee mugs for cups.

1 **pound pork tenderloin, cut into bite-size pieces**	1/4 **cup chopped green bell pepper**
1/2 **cup chopped red onion (fresh or frozen)**	1 **pound quick-cooking, fat-free shredded hash browns**
	1/2 **cup barbeque sauce**

- Coat a 12-inch nonstick skillet with nonfat cooking spray.
- Combine the pork, onion, and bell pepper in a skillet over medium heat. Cook, covered, for 4 to 5 minutes, stirring occasionally.
- Top with shredded hash browns. Cover and cook 6 to 8 minutes longer, stirring occasionally until the meat and potatoes are fully cooked.
- Reduce the heat to low. Add the barbeque sauce. Gently stir until well mixed.
- Serve immediately.

Yield: 4 (1-cup) servings

Calories: 257 (16% fat); Total Fat: 5 gm; Cholesterol: 74 mg; Carbohydrate: 26 gm; Dietary Fiber: 3 gm; Protein: 27 gm; Sodium: 337 mg
Diabetic Exchanges: 2 starch, 3 very lean meat

Preparation time: 5 minutes or less
Cooking time: 15 minutes or less
Total time: 20 minutes or less

Menu Idea: Sassy Slaw (page 91) from *Busy People's Low-Fat Cookbook* tastes excellent with this.

Mushroom & Chicken Skillet Casserole

The flavor of fresh mushrooms in the casserole captures your taste buds.

1	pound skinless, boneless chicken breasts, cut into bite-size pieces	2	cups instant rice
		8	ounces fresh mushrooms, thinly sliced
1	(14-ounce) can fat-free chicken broth	1	(10³/₄-ounce) can 98% fat-free cream of celery soup
½	teaspoon dried thyme		

- In a 12-inch nonstick skillet, cook the chicken in the chicken broth and ¼ cup hot water until the mixture comes to a full boil.
- Stir in the thyme and rice, making sure the rice is covered with the broth.
- Place the mushrooms on top. (The steam will cook the thin slices of mushrooms.)
- Cover the skillet. Turn off the heat and let stand 5 minutes.
- Turn the heat to low and cook for a couple of minutes while gently stirring the soup and mushrooms into the chicken and rice. Continue stirring until the ingredients are well mixed and the entire dish is hot.

Yield: 4 (1½-cup) servings

Calories: 361 (9% fat); Total Fat: 3 gm; Cholesterol: 69 mg; Carbohydrate: 45 gm; Dietary Fiber: 1 gm; Protein: 34 gm; Sodium: 786 mg
Diabetic Exchanges: 3 starch, 3 very lean meat

Preparation time: 10 minutes or less
Cooking time: 10 minutes or less
Total time: 20 minutes or less

Menu Idea: Make this a well-balanced meal by serving Fresh Broccoli Salad (page 53) from *Busy People's Down-Home Cooking Without the Down-Home Fat* with this recipe.

Speedy Sweets

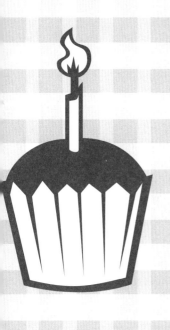

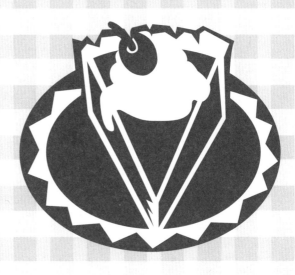

Orange Sugar Cookies

An old-time favorite, these soft, moist cookies are a sure winner with our family!

Cookies:
- 1/3 cup plus 1 tablespoon orange juice
- 1 cup reduced-fat baking mix (I use Bisquick)
- 1/4 cup sugar
- 1 teaspoon orange extract (found next to vanilla extract)

Frosting:
- 2 tablespoons reduced-fat vanilla frosting (I use Betty Crocker Sweet Rewards)
- 2 drops orange extract

- Preheat the oven to 400 degrees. Coat two cookie sheets with nonfat cooking spray.
- In a medium bowl mix all the orange juice, baking mix, sugar, and orange extract together with a spatula until well mixed.
- Drop by rounded teaspoonfuls onto the prepared cookie sheets.
- Bake for 4 minutes or until the bottoms are lightly golden brown.
- While the cookies are baking, microwave the frosting for 15 seconds, just enough to melt it. Stir in the orange extract. Drizzle the frosting over the warm, baked cookies.

Yield: 24 cookies

(Nutritional information per cookie)
Calories: 35 (0% fat); Total Fat: 0 gm; Cholesterol: 0 mg; Carbohydrate: 7 gm; Dietary Fiber: 0 gm; Protein: 0 gm; Sodium: 61 mg
Diabetic Exchanges: 1/2 other carbohydrate

Preparation time: 5 minutes or less
Cooking time: 5 minutes or less
Total time: 10 minutes or less

Sour Cream Cookies

A slight variation to the traditional sugar cookie, these taste very good!

$1/3$ cup plus 1 tablespoon fat-free sour cream	$1/2$ cup powdered sugar
1 cup reduced-fat baking mix (I use Bisquick)	1 tablespoon skim milk
	1 tablespoon granulated sugar

- Preheat the oven to 400 degrees. Coat two cookie sheets with nonfat cooking spray.
- In a medium bowl mix all the sour cream, baking mix, powdered sugar, and milk together with a spatula until well mixed.
- Drop by rounded teaspoonfuls onto the prepared cookie sheets. Sprinkle the tops lightly with the granulated sugar.
- Bake for 5 minutes or until the bottoms are lightly golden brown.

Yield: 24 cookies

(Nutritional information per cookie)
Calories: 35 (8% fat); Total Fat: trace; Cholesterol: 0 mg; Carbohydrate: 7 gm;
Dietary Fiber: 0 gm; Protein: 1 gm; Sodium: 62 mg
Diabetic Exchanges: $1/2$ other carbohydrate

Preparation time: 5 minutes or less
Cooking time: 5 minutes or less
Total time: 10 minutes or less

Coconut Sugar Cookies

These coconut cookies are incredibly delicious!

1 teaspoon imitation coconut extract (I use Durkee, found by the vanilla)	1 cup reduced-fat baking mix (I use Bisquick)
1/3 cup fat-free virgin piña colada mix (I use Lemix)	1/4 cup sugar
	1 1/2 tablespoons shredded coconut

- Preheat the oven to 400 degrees. Coat two cookie sheets with nonfat cooking spray.
- In a medium bowl mix the coconut flavoring, piña colada mix, baking mix, and sugar together with a spoon until well blended.
- Drop by rounded teaspoonfuls onto the prepared cookie sheets.
- Sprinkle the tops of the cookies lightly with the coconut.
- Bake for 4 minutes or until the bottoms are golden brown.

Yield: 24 cookies

(Nutritional information per cookie)
Calories: 32 (14% fat); Total Fat: trace; Cholesterol: 0 mg; Carbohydrate: 6 gm;
Dietary Fiber: 0 gm; Protein: 0 gm; Sodium: 58 mg
Diabetic Exchanges: 1/2 other carbohydrate

Preparation time: 5 minutes or less
Cooking time: 4 minutes or less
Total time: 9 minutes or less

Chocolate Coconut Cookies

These cookies are definitely rated A plus.

1 **(18.25-ounce) box German chocolate super moist cake mix, dry (I use Betty Crocker)**	1 **teaspoon imitation coconut extract (I use Durkee)**
2 **(4-ounce) containers egg substitute (I use Egg Beaters) or 8 egg whites**	**³/4 cup fat-free virgin piña colada mix (I use Lemix)**
	¹/4 cup shredded coconut

- Preheat the oven to 400 degrees. Coat four cookie sheets with nonfat cooking spray.
- Mix the cake mix, egg substitute, coconut extract, and piña colada mix together with a spoon until well blended.
- Drop by rounded teaspoonfuls onto the prepared cookie sheets.
- Sprinkle the tops lightly with the coconut.
- Bake for 4 to 5 minutes or until the bottoms are lightly browned.

Note: You will probably have to bake these two dozen at a time depending on the size of your oven. Cooking time is based on baking two dozen at a time.

Yield: 78 cookies

(Nutritional information per cookie)
Calories: 32 (20% fat); Total Fat: 1 gm; Cholesterol: 0 mg; Carbohydrate: 6 gm;
Dietary Fiber: 0 gm; Protein: 1 gm; Sodium: 46 mg
Diabetic Exchanges: ¹/2 other carbohydrate

Preparation time: 10 minutes or less
Cooking time: 20 minutes or less (5 minutes per two dozen)
Total time: 30 minutes or less

Chocolate Sour Cream Cookies

A chocolate lover's delight, these cookies are delectable!

I	(18.25-ounce) box reduced-fat devil's food cake mix, dry (I use Betty Crocker Sweet Rewards)	2	(4-ounce) containers egg substitute (I use Egg Beaters) or 8 egg whites
		¹/2	cup nonfat sour cream

- Preheat the oven to 400 degrees. Coat four cookie sheets with nonfat cooking spray.
- In a medium bowl stir the cake mix, egg substitute, and sour cream together with a spatula until well mixed.
- Drop by rounded teaspoonfuls onto the prepared cookie sheets.
- Bake for 4 minutes or until the centers of the cookies are set.

Note: Cooking time is based on baking two dozen at a time.

Yield: 78 cookies

(Nutritional information per cookie)
Calories: 30 (17% fat); Total Fat: 1 gm; Cholesterol: 0 mg; Carbohydrate: 6 gm; Dietary Fiber: 0 gm; Protein: 1 gm; Sodium: 57 mg
Diabetic Exchanges: ¹/2 other carbohydrate

Chocolate Coconut Sour Cream Cookies:

Make the recipe the same except stir 1 teaspoon coconut extract into the batter with the other ingredients. Sprinkle with ¹/4 cup shredded coconut before baking.

(Nutritional information per cookie)
Calories: 31 (18% fat); Total Fat: 1 gm; Cholesterol: 0 mg; Carbohydrate: 6 gm; Dietary Fiber: 0 gm; Protein: 1 gm; Sodium: 58 mg
Diabetic Exchanges: ¹/2 other carbohydrate

Preparation time: 10 minutes or less
Cooking time: 16 minutes or less (4 minutes per two dozen)
Total time: 26 minutes or less

Soft Apple Cinnamon Cookies

These cookies have a nice autumn flavor and are a great treat after playing in the leaves!

1/3 cup plus 1 tablespoon skim milk	1 teaspoon ground cinnamon
1 cup reduced-fat baking mix (I use Bisquick)	1 cup chopped Granny Smith apple or any good baking apple (do not use Red Delicious)
1/4 cup packed dark brown sugar	

- Preheat the oven to 400 degrees. Coat two cookie sheets with nonfat cooking spray.
- In a medium bowl, mix all the milk, baking mix, brown sugar, cinnamon, and apple together with a spoon until well mixed.
- Drop by rounded teaspoonfuls onto the prepared cookie sheets.
- Bake for 4 minutes or until lightly golden brown on the bottoms.

Yield: 24 cookies

(Nutritional information per cookie)
Calories: 32 (10% fat); Total Fat: trace; Cholesterol: 0 mg; Carbohydrate: 7 gm;
Dietary Fiber: 0 gm; Protein: 1 gm; Sodium: 61 mg
Diabetic Exchanges: $1/2$ other carbohydrate

Preparation time: 10 minutes or less
Cooking time: 4 minutes or less
Total time: 14 minutes or less

Cappuccino Cookies

These babies are excellent!

I	(18.25-ounce) box reduced-fat devil's food cake mix, dry (I use Betty Crocker Sweet Rewards)	I	teaspoon ground cinnamon
I	tablespoon instant coffee granules	$3/4$	cup skim milk
		2	(4-ounce) containers egg substitute (I use Egg Beaters) or 8 egg whites

- Preheat the oven to 400 degrees. Coat four cookie sheets with nonfat cooking spray.
- In a medium bowl mix the cake mix, instant coffee, cinnamon, milk, and egg substitute together with a spatula until well blended.
- Drop by rounded heaping teaspoonfuls onto the prepared cookie sheets.
- Bake for 5 minutes or until the centers are set.

Note: You will probably have to cook these two dozen at a time depending on the size of your oven. Cooking time is based on cooking two dozen at a time.

Yield: 48 cookies

(Nutritional information per cookie)
Calories: 47 (17% fat); Total Fat: 1 gm; Cholesterol: 0 mg; Carbohydrate: 9 gm; Dietary Fiber: 0 gm; Protein: 1 gm; Sodium: 93 mg
Diabetic Exchanges: $1/2$ other carbohydrate

Amaretto Cappuccino Cookies:
Make the Cappuccino Cookies recipe exactly the same and stir in 2 teaspoons almond extract.

(Nutritional information per cookie)
Calories: 48 (17% fat); Total Fat: 1 gm; Cholesterol: 0 mg; Carbohydrate: 9 gm; Dietary Fiber: 0 gm; Protein: 1 gm; Sodium: 93 mg
Diabetic Exchanges: $1/2$ other carbohydrate

Preparation time: 10 minutes or less
Cooking time: 10 minutes or less (5 minutes per two dozen)
Total time: 20 minutes or less

Delicious Date Cookies

I hit a "bull's-eye" when I created these! The recipe title says it all. I love the flavor combination.

$1/3$ cup plus I tablespoon orange juice	$1/4$ cup packed dark brown sugar
I cup reduced-fat baking mix (I use Bisquick)	I teaspoon ground cinnamon
	$1/2$ cup chopped dates (I use Dole brand, found in baking section)

- Preheat the oven to 400 degrees. Coat two cookie sheets with nonfat cooking spray.
- In a medium bowl mix all the orange juice, baking mix, brown sugar, cinnamon, and dates together with a spoon until well mixed.
- Drop by rounded teaspoonfuls onto the prepared cookie sheets.
- Bake for 5 minutes or until lightly brown on the bottoms.

Note: These are also good with cranberries or raisins instead of dates. Simply substitute $1/2$ cup cranberries or raisins for the dates.

Yield: 24 cookies

(Nutritional information per cookie)
(with dates) Calories: 40 (0% fat); Total Fat: 0 gm; Cholesterol: 0 mg; Carbohydrate: 9 gm; Dietary Fiber: 0 gm; Protein: 1 gm; Sodium: 59 mg
Diabetic Exchanges: $1/2$ other carbohydrate
(with cranberries) Calories: 38 (0% fat); Total Fat: 0 gm; Cholesterol: 0 mg; Carbohydrate: 8 gm; Dietary Fiber: 0 gm; Protein: 0 gm; Sodium: 59 mg
Diabetic Exchanges: $1/2$ other carbohydrate
(with raisins) Calories: 40 (0% fat); Total Fat: 0 gm; Cholesterol: 0 mg; Carbohydrate: 9 gm; Dietary Fiber: 0 gm; Protein: 1 gm; Sodium: 60 mg
Diabetic Exchanges: $1/2$ other carbohydrate

Preparation time: 10 minutes or less
Cooking time: 5 minutes or less
Total time: 15 minutes or less

Very Vanilla Cookies

These are very simple and very easy. If you like sugar cookies, you'll like these.

1/3 cup plus I tablespoon skim milk	I teaspoon vanilla extract
I cup reduced-fat baking mix (I use Bisquick)	2 tablespoons reduced-fat vanilla frosting (I use Betty Crocker Sweet Rewards)
1/4 cup sugar	

- Preheat the oven to 400 degrees. Coat two cookie sheets with nonfat cooking spray.
- Combine all the milk, baking mix, sugar, and vanilla together in a medium bowl with a spoon until well mixed.
- Drop by rounded teaspoonfuls onto the prepared cookie sheets.
- Bake for 4 minutes or until lightly golden brown on the bottoms.
- Microwave the frosting for 10 to 15 seconds, just enough to melt it. Drizzle the frosting over the cookies.

Note: These are also good with a couple drops of almond extract added to the frosting before microwaving. The nutritional information is the same.

Yield: 24 cookies

(Nutritional information per cookie)
Calories: 34 (12% fat); Total Fat: trace; Cholesterol: 0 mg; Carbohydrate: 7 gm; Dietary Fiber: 0 gm; Protein: 1 gm; Sodium: 63 mg
Diabetic Exchanges: 1/2 other carbohydrate

Preparation time: 10 minutes or less
Cooking time: 4 minutes or less
Total time: 14 minutes or less

Citrus Spice Cookies

Soft, fragrant, and flavorful, these cookies are a good accompaniment for hot tea.

1/2 teaspoon ground cinnamon	1/3 cup plus 1 tablespoon orange juice
1/4 cup packed dark brown sugar	
1 cup reduced-fat baking mix (I use Bisquick)	

- Preheat the oven to 400 degrees. Coat two cookie sheets with nonfat cooking spray.
- In a medium bowl combine the cinnamon, brown sugar, baking mix, and all the orange juice together with a spoon until well mixed.
- Drop by rounded teaspoonfuls onto the prepared cookie sheets.
- Bake for 4 minutes or until the bottoms are lightly golden brown.

Yield: 24 cookies

(Nutritional information per cookie)
Calories: 30 (10% fat): Total Fat: trace; Cholesterol: 0 mg; Carbohydrate: 6 gm; Dietary Fiber: 0 gm; Protein: 0 gm; Sodium: 59 mg
Diabetic Exchanges: 1/2 other carbohydrate

Preparation time: 10 minutes or less
Cooking time: 4 minutes or less
Total time: 14 minutes or less

Pistachio Cookies

The pretty "spring green" color makes these perfect to serve on Easter or St. Patrick's Day.

¹/₃ cup plus 1 tablespoon water	¹/₄ cup plus 1 tablespoon sugar
1 cup reduced-fat baking mix (I use Bisquick)	1 egg white
1 (1-ounce) box pistachio fat-free sugar-free instant pudding, dry (I use Jell-O)	¹/₂ teaspoon almond extract

- Preheat the oven to 350 degrees. Coat two cookie sheets with nonfat cooking spray.
- In a medium bowl combine all the water, baking mix, instant pudding, ¹/₄ cup of the sugar, egg white, and almond extract together with a spoon until well mixed.
- Drop by rounded teaspoonfuls onto the prepared cookie sheets. Evenly sprinkle the cookies with the remaining 1 tablespoon sugar.
- Bake for 8 minutes or until the bottoms are lightly golden brown.

Yield: 24 cookies

(Nutritional information per cookie)
Calories: 34 (9% fat); Total Fat: trace; Cholesterol: 0 mg; Carbohydrate: 7 gm;
Dietary Fiber: 0 gm; Protein: 1 gm; Sodium: 109 mg
Diabetic Exchanges: ¹/₂ other carbohydrate

Preparation time: 10 minutes or less
Cooking time: 8 minutes or less
Total time: 18 minutes or less

Chocolate Chewy Cookies

Gloria Pitzer, author of The Recipe Detective, *published a high-fat version of this recipe and I converted it to an almost fat-free cookie. I give her all the credit for creating this delicious cookie, which she states reminds her of the kind Mrs. Field's used to have. Thank you, Gloria, for this wonderful cookie idea!*

1	(8-ounce) container fat-free whipped topping (I use Cool Whip Free)	1	(18.25-ounce) box reduced-fat chocolate cake mix, dry (I use Betty Crocker Sweet Rewards)
2	egg whites	1/4	cup powdered sugar

- Preheat the oven to 350 degrees. Coat two cookie sheets with nonfat cooking spray.
- Beat the whipped topping in a medium mixing bowl until smooth. Add the egg whites and mix well.
- Stir in the cake mix until completely mixed.
- Dip rounded tablespoonfuls of cookie dough into the powdered sugar.
- Place each cookie covered with powdered sugar onto the prepared cookie sheets. Bake for 10 minutes or until set but not brown.
- Let cool for a few minutes on the cookie sheets, then transfer to wax paper.

Note: You can substitute lemon cake mix or carrot cake mix for the chocolate for variations. Add 1 calorie more per cookie for these variations.

Yield: 58 cookies

(Nutritional information per cookie)
Calories: 46 (16% fat); Total Fat: 1 gm; Cholesterol: 0 mg; Carbohydrate: 9 gm; Dietary Fiber: 0 gm; Protein: 0 gm; Sodium: 59 mg
Diabetic Exchanges: 1/2 other carbohydrate

Preparation time: 10 minutes or less
Cooking time: 20 minutes or less (10 minutes per two dozen)
Total time: 30 minutes or less

Sugar-Free Lemon Meringue Cookies

Simply substitute 1 teaspoon of your favorite flavored extracts, such as vanilla, maple, coconut, or almond, in place of the lemon extract. The nutritional information stays the same. These cookies need to be eaten the day they are made.

3 egg whites	1/4 teaspoon cream of tartar
3/4 cup Splenda Granular	1 teaspoon lemon extract

- Preheat the oven to 350 degrees.
- Coat a cookie sheet with nonfat cooking spray.
- In a large glass mixing bowl beat the egg whites with an electric mixer for 3 to 4 minutes or until stiff peaks form, which is when you lift the mixer up (after the mixer is turned off) and the little mountain peaks keep their shape.
- Slowly add the Splenda, cream of tartar, and lemon extract into the egg whites, continuously beating with the mixer until well blended.
- Drop by heaping tablespoonfuls onto the prepared cookie sheet, scraping the meringue out of the measuring spoon with the back of another spoon. You will be able to put all 15 meringues onto one cookie sheet.
- Bake for 8 minutes or until golden brown on the tops and bottoms of the cookies.
- Cookies may become slightly smaller in size as they cool; however, they should not go flat. If they become flat, then your egg whites were not beaten enough.

Note: Do not use plastic bowl when beating the egg whites. Stiff peaks will not form in a plastic bowl.

Yield: 15 cookies

(Nutritional information is per cookie.)
Calories: 9 (0% fat); Total Fat: 0 gm; Cholesterol: 0 mg; Carbohydrate: 1 gm; Dietary Fiber: 0 gm; Protein: 1 gm; Sodium: 11 mg
Diabetic Exchanges: Free

Preparation time: 15 minutes or less
Cooking time: 8 minutes or less
Total time: 23 minutes or less

Double Chocolate Graham Cookies

Isn't it amazing that a double chocolate cookie can be diabetic too! It's good and good for you.

3	egg whites	1	tablespoon cocoa powder
1	cup Splenda Granular	1/2	cup graham cracker crumbs
1/4	teaspoon cream of tartar	2	tablespoons mini chocolate chips
1	teaspoon vanilla extract		

- Preheat the oven to 350 degrees.
- Coat a cookie sheet with nonfat cooking spray.
- In a large glass mixing bowl (stiff peaks will not form in a plastic bowl) with an electric mixer, beat the egg whites for 3 to 4 minutes or until stiff peaks form, which is when you lift the mixer up (after the mixer is turned off) and the peaks keep their shape.
- Slowly add the Splenda, cream of tartar, vanilla extract, and cocoa powder into the egg whites, continuously beating with the mixer until well blended.
- Scrape off as much of the egg mixture as you can from the beaters. Set the mixer aside.
- Using a rubber spatula, fold in the graham cracker crumbs and chocolate chips until well mixed. (To "fold" is a cooking term that means to very gently lift from the bottom of the batter and stir.)
- Drop by heaping tablespoonfuls onto the prepared cookie sheet, scraping the dough out of the measuring spoon with the back of another spoon. You will be able to put all 15 cookies onto one cookie sheet.
- Bake for 8 minutes or until golden brown on the top and bottom of the cookies.

Note: To keep the cookies moist, store them on a plate inside of a sealed zip-top plastic bag with a slice of bread.

Yield: 15 (1-cookie) servings

(Nutritional information per cookie)
Calories: 31 (21% fat); Total Fat: 1 gm; Cholesterol: 0 mg; Carbohydrate: 5 gm;
Dietary Fiber: 0 gm; Protein: 1 gm; Sodium: 28 mg
Diabetic Exchanges: $1/2$ other carbohydrate

Preparation time: 10 minutes or less
Cooking time: 8 minutes or less
Total time: 18 minutes or less

Coconut Cookies

These cookies are one of my favorites.

4 egg whites	2 cups crushed unsweetened whole wheat cereal flakes
1 cup Splenda Granular	
1½ teaspoons imitation coconut flavoring	2 tablespoons plus 2 tablespoons shredded coconut
2 cups unsweetened puffed rice cereal	

- Coat two cookie sheets with nonfat cooking spray. Set aside.
- In a medium glass bowl, beat the egg whites until frothy with an electric mixer on medium-high speed.
- Slowly add the Splenda a few tablespoons at a time. (You may want to turn the mixer off when adding Splenda to help prevent Splenda from flying all over.) Continue beating until all of the Splenda is used. Beat in the coconut flavoring with the mixer until well blended.
- Gently stir in the puffed rice cereal, the crushed cereal flakes, and 2 tablespoons of the coconut with a spatula.
- Drop by rounded tablespoonfuls onto the prepared cookie sheets, using a knife to scrape the dough out of the spoon.
- Lightly sprinkle the remaining 2 tablespoons coconut evenly over the entire batch of cookies.
- Bake for 12 to 14 minutes or until the cookies are light brown around the edges.

Yield: 20 (1-cookie) servings

(Nutritional information per cookie)
Calories: 35 (12% fat); Total Fat: 1 gm; Cholesterol: 0 mg; Carbohydrate: 7 gm; Dietary Fiber: 0 gm; Protein: 1 gm; Sodium: 60 mg
Diabetic Exchanges: ½ other carbohydrate

Preparation time: 10 minutes or less
Cooking time: 14 minutes or less
Total time: 24 minutes or less

Crunchy Kisses (Cookies)

Expect these crunchy cookies to go fast.

2 egg whites	2½ cups unsweetened whole wheat cereal flakes, crushed
1 cup Splenda Granular	
1 teaspoon vanilla extract	

- Preheat the oven to 350 degrees.
- Coat two cookie sheets with nonfat cooking spray.
- In a medium glass bowl beat the egg whites with an electric mixer on medium-high speed until frothy.
- Slowly add the Splenda a few tablespoons at a time. (You may want to turn the mixer off when adding Splenda to help prevent Splenda from flying all over.) Continue beating until all of the Splenda is used. Beat in the vanilla with a mixer until well blended.
- Gently stir in the cereal with a spatula.
- Drop by rounded teaspoonfuls onto the prepared cookie sheets, using a knife to scrape the dough out of the spoon. You can put twenty cookies on one cookie sheet.
- Bake for 12 to 15 minutes or until cookies are light brown around the edges.

Yield: 8 (5-cookie) servings

Calories: 55 (0% fat); Total Fat: 0 gm; Cholesterol:0 mg; Carbohydrate: 10 gm; Dietary Fiber: 0 gm; Protein: 3 gm; Sodium: 84 mg
Diabetic Exchanges: ½ other carbohydrate

Preparation time: 10 minutes or less
Cooking time: 15 minutes or less
Total time: 25 minutes or less

Crunchy Chocolate Kisses (Cookies)

You're gonna love these!

2 egg whites	2 cups unsweetened cereal flakes, crushed (I use Special K)
1 cup Splenda Granular	2 tablespoons mini chocolate chips
1 tablespoon cocoa powder	

- Preheat the oven to 350 degrees.
- Coat two cookie sheets with nonfat cooking spray. Set aside.
- In a medium glass bowl beat the egg whites until frothy with an electric mixer on medium-high speed.
- Slowly add the Splenda a few tablespoons at a time. (You may want to turn the mixer off when adding Splenda to help prevent Splenda from flying all over.) Continue beating until all of the Splenda is added. Beat in the cocoa powder until well blended.
- Gently stir in the cereal with a spatula.
- Drop by rounded teaspoonfuls onto the prepared cookie sheets, using a knife to scrape the dough out of the spoon. You can put twenty cookies on one cookie sheet.
- Sprinkle 5 mini chocolate chips on top of each cookie.
- Bake for 12 to 15 minutes or until the cookies are light brown around the edges.

Yield: 8 (5-cookie) servings

Calories: 61 (14% fat); Total Fat: 1 gm; Cholesterol: 0 mg; Carbohydrate: 11 gm; Dietary Fiber: 1 gm; Protein: 3 gm; Sodium: 70 mg
Diabetic Exchanges: $1/2$ other carbohydrate

Preparation time: 10 minutes or less
Cooking time: 15 minutes or less
Total time: 25 minutes or less

Butterscotch Crunchy Kisses (Cookies)

These are almost like eating sweet, crunchy candy.

3 egg whites	2 1/2 cups crushed unsweetened cereal flakes(I use Special K)
1/3 cup Splenda Granular	1/4 cup finely chopped butterscotch chips
1 (1-ounce) box sugar-free, fat-free instant butterscotch pudding mix (Do not make as directed on box)	

- Preheat the oven to 350 degrees.
- Coat two cookie sheets with nonfat cooking spray.
- In a medium glass bowl beat the egg whites with an electric mixer on medium-high speed until frothy.
- Slowly add the Splenda a few tablespoons at a time. (You may want to turn the mixer off when adding Splenda to help prevent Splenda from flying all over.) Continue beating until all of the Splenda is added. Beat in the pudding mix until well blended.
- Gently stir in the cereal with a spatula.
- Drop by rounded teaspoonfuls onto the prepared cookie sheets, using a knife to scrape the dough out of the spoon. You can put 25 cookies on one cookie sheet.
- Lightly and evenly sprinkle the chopped butterscotch chips over the entire batch of cookies.
- Bake for 12 to 15 minutes or until the cookies are light brown around the edges.

Yield: 9 (5-cookie) servings

Calories: 87 (21% fat); Total Fat: 2 gm; Cholesterol: 0 mg; Carbohydrate: 14 gm; Dietary Fiber: 0 gm; Protein: 3 gm; Sodium: 217 mg
Diabetic Exchanges: 1 other carbohydrate

Preparation time: 10 minutes or less
Cooking time: 15 minutes or less
Total time: 25 minutes or less

Chocolate Cherry Cookie Squares

The flavor combination is a true winner! These cookies taste a lot like super light brownies with cherry pieces in them.

1/3 cup cocoa powder	1/2 cup water
1 teaspoon almond extract	1 (16-ounce) box angel food cake mix, dry
1/3 cup reduced-fat baking mix (I use Bisquick)	10 maraschino cherries, cut into eighths*
1/3 cup egg substitute (I use Egg Beaters) or 3 egg whites	

- Preheat the oven to 350 degrees.
- Coat an 11 x 17-inch jelly roll pan with nonfat cooking spray.
- In a medium bowl mix together the cocoa powder, almond extract, baking mix, egg substitute, water, cake mix, and maraschino cherries with an electric mixer on medium-low speed. Increase the speed to high until well mixed. (The batter will be thick and doughy.)
- Spread into the prepared pan with a smooth-edged knife that has been sprayed with nonfat cooking spray. It may take up to 4 or 5 minutes to spread out because the dough is thick and sticky. Take your time and it will evenly cover the entire pan.
- Bake for 10 minutes.
- Cool. Cut into forty 2-inch squares.

Note: To cut the cherries into eighths, cut in half diagonally. Turn and cut in half again. Turn onto the side and cut through all four pieces at once. To keep cookies moist store on a plate inside of a sealed zip-top plastic bag with a slice of bread.

Yield 40 (1-square) servings

Calories: 52 (0% fat); Total Fat: 0 gm; Cholesterol: 0 mg; Carbohydrate: 11 gm; Dietary Fiber: 0 gm; Protein: 1 gm; Sodium: 114 mg
Diabetic Exchanges: 1/2 other carbohydrate

Preparation time: 10 minutes or less
Cooking time: 10 minutes or less
Total time: 20 minutes or less

Piña Colada Cookie Squares

The tropical flavors of the coconut and pineapple together remind me of Hawaii. Wouldn't you love to be there? Me too!

1 (16-ounce) box angel food cake mix, dry	1 teaspoon coconut extract
1/2 cup egg substitute (I use Egg Beaters) or 4 egg whites	1 1/4 cups crushed pineapple in unsweetened juice*
1 cup reduced-fat baking mix (I use Bisquick)	1/4 cup shredded coconut

- Preheat the oven to 350 degrees.
- Coat an 11 x 17-inch jelly roll pan with nonfat cooking spray.
- In a medium bowl mix together the cake mix, egg substitute, baking mix, coconut extract, and pineapple with an electric mixer on medium-low speed.
- Spread into the prepared pan with a smooth-edged knife that has been sprayed with nonfat cooking spray.
- Lightly sprinkle the shredded coconut evenly over the top of the batter.
- Bake for 10 minutes.
- Let cool and cut into forty 2-inch squares.

*Note: Use a 20-ounce can of crushed pineapple. Squeeze out or drain 1½ cups pineapple juice. Discard juice. Use only the crushed pineapple, which will measure 1¼ cups.

Yield: 40 (1-square) servings

Calories: 62 (0% fat); Total Fat: 0 gm; Cholesterol: 0 mg; Carbohydrate: 13 gm; Dietary Fiber: 0 gm; Protein: 1 gm; Sodium: 142 mg
Diabetic Exchanges: 1 other carbohydrate

Preparation time: 10 minutes or less
Cooking time: 10 minutes or less
Total time: 20 minutes or less

Chocolate Mint Cookie Squares

Cookie Squares are drier and firmer than a Cookie-Snack Cake Square. Cookie Squares only take ten minutes to bake and they are about two inches square. That's a nice size cookie made up fast! Over three dozen homemade cookies completely done from start to finish in twenty minutes or less!

1/3 cup cocoa powder	1/2 cup water
1 teaspoon mint extract	1 (16-ounce) box angel food cake
1/3 cup reduced-fat baking mix (I use Bisquick)	mix, dry
	1/3 cup mini chocolate chips
1/2 cup egg substitute (I use Egg Beaters) or 4 egg whites	

- Preheat the oven to 350 degrees.
- Coat an 11 x 17-inch jelly roll pan with nonfat cooking spray.
- In a medium bowl mix together the cocoa powder, mint extract, baking mix, egg substitute, water, and cake mix with an electric mixer on medium-low speed. Increase the speed to high until well mixed. (The batter will be super thick and doughy.)
- Spread into the prepared pan with a smooth-edged knife that has been sprayed with nonfat cooking spray. This is the most time-consuming part of preparing this recipe because the dough is thick and sticky. It may take up to 4 or 5 minutes to spread out. Trust me, take your time and it will evenly cover the entire bottom the pan.
- Sprinkle evenly with the chocolate chips.
- Bake for 10 minutes.
- Cool. Cut into forty 2-inch squares.

Note: To keep cookies moist store on a plate inside of a sealed zip-top plastic bag with a slice of bread.

Yield 40 (1-square) servings

Calories: 57 (9% fat); Total Fat: 1 gm; Cholesterol: 0 mg; Carbohydrate: 11 gm; Dietary Fiber: 0 gm; Protein: 2 gm; Sodium: 117 mg
Diabetic Exchanges: 1 other carbohydrate

Preparation time: 10 minutes or less
Cooking time: 10 minutes or less
Total time: 20 minutes or less

Cherry Cookie Snack Cake Squares

Okay, so the title of this recipe is pretty long. But when you taste them you'll see how they got their name. These tasty treats are a cross between a cookie and a snack cake.

1 (16-ounce) box angel food cake mix, dry	1 cup reduced-fat baking mix (I use Bisquick)
1 (20-ounce) can light cherry pie filling	

- Preheat the oven to 350 degrees.
- Coat an 11 x 17-inch jelly roll pan with nonfat cooking spray.
- Mix the cake mix, pie filling, and baking mix together with a spatula in a medium bowl until well mixed.
- Spread the thick batter into the prepared pan.
- Bake for 10 minutes.
- Cool a couple of minutes before cutting into forty 2-inch squares. These are really good served warm, too!

Yield: 40 (1-square) servings

Calories: 59 (0% fat); Total Fat: 0 gm; Cholesterol: 0 mg; Carbohydrate: 13 gm; Dietary Fiber: 0 gm; Protein: 1 gm; Sodium: 135 mg
Diabetic Exchanges: 1 other carbohydrate

Preparation time: 5 minutes or less
Cooking time: 10 minutes or less
Total time: 15 minutes or less

Cappuccino Snack Cake

This cake tastes delicious! It's rich, smooth, and moist!

1 (18.25-ounce) package devil's food super moist cake mix, dry (I use Betty Crocker)	1 tablespoon instant coffee granules
1¹/₃ cups water	1 teaspoon ground cinnamon, plus extra for topping (optional)
4 egg whites	¹/₂ cup applesauce

- Preheat the oven to 350 degrees. Coat three 9-inch square cake pans with nonfat cooking spray.
- In a mixing bowl beat the cake mix, water, egg whites, instant coffee, cinnamon, and applesauce on low speed for 1 minute, scraping the bowl constantly. (Or stir by hand for 2 minutes.) Divide the batter evenly into the prepared pans.
- Bake for 15 to 20 minutes or until a toothpick inserted in the center comes out clean.
- Cool the cakes for 10 minutes in the pan. Sprinkle lightly with cinnamon, if desired. Cut each pan into 9 squares.

Yield: 27 servings

Calories: 83 (19% fat); Total Fat: 2 gm; Cholesterol: 0 mg; Carbohydrate: 15 gm; Dietary Fiber: 1 gm; Protein: 1 gm; Sodium: 154 mg
Diabetic Exchanges: 1 other carbohydrate

Preparation time: 10 minutes or less
Cooking time: 20 minutes or less
Total time: 30 minutes or less

Double Chocolate Sour Cream Snack Cake

This cake is guaranteed to curb any chocolate sweet tooth.

1 (18.25-ounce) box reduced-fat devil's food cake mix, dry (I use Betty Crocker Sweet Rewards)

2 (4-ounce) containers egg substitute (I use Egg Beaters) or 8 egg whites

1/2 cup fat-free sour cream

1/4 cup reduced-fat chocolate frosting (I use Betty Crocker Sweet Rewards)

- Preheat the oven to 350 degrees. Coat an 11 x 17-inch jelly roll pan with nonfat cooking spray.
- Mix the cake mix, egg substitute, and sour cream together in a medium bowl with a spatula until well mixed.
- Spread into the prepared pan.
- Bake for 15 minutes.
- Microwave the frosting for 15 to 25 seconds or until melted. Drizzle over the snack cake.

Note: For a Double Chocolate Sour Cream Coconut Snack Cake, stir 1 teaspoon coconut extract into the batter and after spreading the batter into the prepared pan, sprinkle with ¼ cup shredded coconut.

Yield: 30 squares

(Nutritional information per square)
(without coconut) Calories: 80 (9% fat); Total Fat: 1 gm; Cholesterol: 0 mg; Carbohydrate: 17 gm; Dietary Fiber: 0 gm; Protein: 2 gm; Sodium: 172 mg
Diabetic Exchanges: 1 other carbohydrate
(with coconut) Calories: 84 (11% fat); Total Fat: 1 gm; Cholesterol: 0 mg; Carbohydrate: 17 gm; Dietary Fiber: 1 gm; Protein: 2 gm; Sodium: 174 mg
Diabetic Exchanges: 1 other carbohydrate

Preparation time: 5 minutes or less
Cooking time: 15 minutes
Total time: 20 minutes or less

Cinnamon Oatmeal Mounds

These healthy treats are good to eat for breakfast on the run. They are shaped in little mounds and are just the right size for curbing your sweet tooth in a nutritious way. They have the flavor and texture of granola and a health food-type cookie combined. They remind me a lot of the granola bites that come individually packaged as a health food.

2 egg whites	3/4 cup crushed Life cereal
1/2 cup Splenda Granular	1 cup crushed Special K cereal
1 teaspoon vanilla extract	1 cup whole grain oatmeal
1/2 teaspoon ground cinnamon	

- Preheat the oven to 350 degrees.
- Coat two cookie sheets with nonfat cooking spray.
- In a large glass bowl beat the egg whites with an electric mixer on high for about 1 minute or until soft peaks form.
- Add the Splenda, vanilla, and cinnamon and continue beating on low until well mixed.
- Pour the crushed cereal into the egg mixture along with the oatmeal. Stir all the ingredients together with a spatula until well mixed.
- Spoon the dough, 1 tablespoonful at a time, onto the prepared cookie sheets.
- Bake for 10 to 12 minutes or until lightly browned on the bottom.

Note: Add chopped raisins or chopped dates if desired; but remember that both are high in natural sugars, so use only a little.

Yield: 21 (1-cookie) servings (without raisins or dates)

Calories: 46 (12% fat); Total Fat: 1 gm; Cholesterol:0 mg; Carbohydrate: 8 gm; Dietary Fiber: 1 gm; Protein: 2 gm; Sodium: 24 mg
Diabetic Exchanges: 1/2 starch

Preparation time: 10 minutes or less
Cooking time: 12 minutes or less
Total time: 22 minutes or less

Creamy Rice Pudding

This is a terrific way to use leftover white rice.

2 (1-ounce) boxes sugar-free instant vanilla pudding mix, dry (I use Jell-O)	1/2 (8-ounce) container fat-free whipped topping, thawed (I use Cool Whip Free)
3 1/2 cups cold skim milk	1 teaspoon almond extract
	1 cup raisins
	2 cups cooked white rice

- In a medium-large bowl briskly whisk together the pudding mix and milk for 2 minutes.
- Stir in the whipped topping, almond extract, raisins, and rice. Keep stirring until well mixed.
- Serve as is or keep chilled until ready to eat.
- If desired, sprinkle top very lightly with ground cinnamon before serving.

Yield: 15 (1/2-cup) servings

Calories: 112 (0% fat); Total Fat: 0 gm; Cholesterol: 1 mg; Carbohydrate: 24 gm; Dietary Fiber: 1 gm; Protein: 3 gm; Sodium: 107 mg
Diabetic Exchanges: 1/2 starch, 1/2 skim milk, 1/2 fruit

Preparation time: 10 minutes or less

Orange Creamsicle Pudding

This recipe was sent in by Cathy West. Thank you, Cathy! It is yummy!

1 (8-ounce) package fat-free cream cheese, softened	1/4 teaspoon vanilla extract
1 (8-ounce) fat-free, sugar-free orange yogurt	1 (0.3-ounce) package orange sugar-free gelatin, dry
5 individual packets Splenda	1 cup fat-free whipped topping (I use Cool Whip Free)

- In a mixing bowl beat the cream cheese and yogurt together with an electric mixer until creamy.
- Add the Splenda and vanilla, then add in the gelatin and mix well.
- Fold in the whipped topping and spoon into four dessert dishes.

Yield: 4 (³⁄₄-cup) servings

Calories: 134 (0% fat); Total Fat: 0 gm; Cholesterol: 11 mg; Carbohydrate: 17 gm;
Dietary Fiber: 0 gm; Protein: 11 gm; Sodium: 378 mg
Diabetic Exchanges: 1 skim milk

Preparation time: 10 minutes

Butterscotch Poppy Seed Cake

This cake is good just as it is for a snack cake. However, I think it tastes best when served warm with a dollop of Butterscotch Cream Dessert Dip (page 266).

I (18.25-ounce) box white cake mix, dry (I use Betty Crocker Super Moist)	4 egg whites or $^1/_2$ cup egg substitute (I use Egg Beaters)
$^1/_4$ cup poppy seeds	$^2/_3$ cup applesauce
I (I-ounce) package sugar-free butterscotch instant pudding(do not make as directed)	I cup water

- Preheat the oven to 350 degrees.
- Coat an 11 x 17-inch jelly roll pan with nonfat cooking spray.
- Mix the cake mix, poppy seeds, pudding mix, egg whites, applesauce, and water together until well mixed.
- Spread in the prepared jelly roll pan.
- Bake for 18 to 23 minutes or until a toothpick inserted in the center comes out clean.
- Let cool a few minutes before cutting if you want to serve it warm. It also tastes good served at room temperature.

Note: Substitute sugar-free, fat-free banana cream instant pudding for the butterscotch pudding for a Banana Poppy Seed Cake.

Yield: 24 servings

(with butterscotch pudding) Calories: 108 (23% fat); Total Fat: 3 gm; Cholesterol: 0 mg; Carbohydrate: 19 gm; Dietary Fiber: 1 gm; Protein: 2 gm; Sodium: 195 mg Diabetic Exchanges: 1$^1/_2$ other carbohydrate, $^1/_2$ fat
(with banana pudding) Calories: 76 (0% fat); Total Fat: 0 gm; Cholesterol: 0 mg; Carbohydrate: 17 gm; Dietary Fiber: 1 gm; Protein: 2 gm; Sodium: 165 mg Diabetic Exchanges: 1 other carbohydrate

Preparation time: 5 minutes or less
   Cooking time: 23 minutes or less
   Total time: 28 minutes or less

Creamsicle Sponge Cake

You can substitute other gelatin flavors for a variation. Try it with strawberry, lime, lemon, or raspberry flavored gelatin and garnish with slices of the respective fruit.

1	(10.5-ounce) angel food cake, cut into 1-inch pieces	1	cup caffeine-free diet Mountain Dew
1	cup fat-free cottage cheese	1	cup fat-free whipped topping (I use Cool Whip Free)
6	individual packets Splenda		Mandarin orange segments for garnish (optional)
2	(0.32-ounce) boxes sugar-free orange gelatin, dry		
2	cups boiling water		

- Coat a 9 x 13 pan with nonfat cooking spray.
- Arrange the cake pieces in the pan. Set aside.
- In a medium bowl beat the cottage cheese and Splenda together with an electric mixer on high for 2 to 3 minutes or until smooth and creamy, scraping the bowl often. Set aside.
- In a separate bowl dissolve both envelopes of the gelatin into the boiling water. Stir until dissolved.
- Pour 1½ cups of the gelatin liquid into the creamed cottage cheese. Beat on low speed until well mixed.
- Pour evenly over the cake pieces in the pan and press the cake pieces firmly into the gelatin with a spatula to help them absorb the gelatin. Once the gelatin is absorbed, smooth the top of the cake evenly with the spatula.
- Pour the soda into the remaining ½ cup gelatin and stir until well mixed. Pour and spread evenly over the cake mixture.
- Cover and refrigerate 3 hours. Serve chilled topped with the whipped topping.
- If desired, garnish with mandarin orange segments.

Yield: 15 servings

Calories: 76 (0% fat); Total Fat: 0 gm; Cholesterol: 1 mg; Carbohydrate: 14 gm; Dietary Fiber: 0 gm; Protein: 4 gm; Sodium: 236 mg
Diabetic Exchanges: 1 other carbohydrate

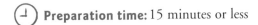 **Preparation time:** 15 minutes or less

Strawberry Shortcake Ice Cream Cake

This delicious summertime treat is especially sweet served on a scorching hot day with freshly picked strawberries!

32	reduced-fat vanilla wafers, crushed	12	large strawberries, cut into thin slices
½	gallon fat-free, sugar-free strawberry frozen yogurt, softened	⅓	cup Splenda Granular
		16	tablespoons fat-free, whipped topping (I use Cool Whip)

- Set aside ½ cup of the cookie crumbs.
- Sprinkle the remaining crumbs onto the bottom of a 9 x 13-inch glass baking dish.
- Spread the frozen yogurt over the crumbs.
- Sprinkle the remaining cookie crumbs over the frozen yogurt.
- Arrange the strawberry slices over the top of the frozen yogurt and cookie crumbs.
- Sprinkle the Splenda over the strawberry slices.
- Place 1 tablespoon dabs of the whipped topping in four rows of four (one dab per serving once cut).
- Cover and freeze until ready to serve.
- Once frozen, let the cake sit out for about 5 minutes before cutting so it is easier to cut through and serve. Cut with a very sharp knife that has been dipped in hot water for cutting ease.

Yield: 16 servings

Calories: 104 (14% fat); Total Fat: 2 gm; Cholesterol: 5 mg; Carbohydrate: 18 gm; Dietary Fiber: 0 gm; Protein: 3 gm; Sodium: 69 mg
Diabetic Exchanges: 1 other carbohydrate, ½ fat

Preparation time: 15 minutes or less

Piña Colada Cake

This cake unites the tropical flavors of the Hawaiian Islands with the comfort foods of down-home cooking for a creative twist to what is normally thought of as a jelly roll cake. However, there is no jelly in this cake.

- 1 (20-ounce) can crushed pineapple in its own juice, drain 1 cup juice and discard
- 1½ teaspoons plus ½ teaspoon coconut extract
- 1 (16-ounce) box angel food cake mix, dry
- 1 (0.9-ounce) box sugar-free fat-free banana cream pudding mix, dry
- 1½ cups skim milk
- 1 (8-ounce) container fat-free whipped topping (I use Cool Whip)
- Lightly toasted shredded coconut (optional)

- Preheat the oven to 350 degrees.
- Line an 11 x 17-inch jelly roll pan with parchment paper. Set aside.
- Stir the crushed pineapple and 1½ teaspoons of the coconut extract together until well mixed in a large bowl.
- Stir in the angel food cake mix until all the ingredients are well mixed. (Batter will poof up in size.)
- Spread the batter into the prepared jelly roll pan.
- Bake for 15 to 20 minutes or until a toothpick inserted in the center comes out clean.
- While the cake bakes, prepare the topping. In a large bowl beat the pudding mix, milk, and remaining ½ teaspoon coconut extract together with an electric mixer on medium speed for 2 minutes.
- Gently fold the whipped topping into the pudding with a spatula until well blended. Keep refrigerated until ready to use.
- Once the cake is finished baking, remove it from the pan and let it cool on a wire baking rack in the refrigerator for about 10 minutes or so to speed up the cooling process.

- While the cake is cooling, broil the coconut on a cookie sheet on the top shelf of the oven for a minute or two, just enough to make the coconut light golden in color.
- Place the cooled cake on a large flat serving platter or back into the cooled jelly roll pan.
- Spread the cream topping over the cooled cake.
- Sprinkle the top very lightly with the toasted shredded coconut, if desired.
- Keep chilled until ready to eat.

Yield: 24 servings

(Nutritional information does not include coconut)
Calories: 103 (0% fat); Total Fat: 0 gm; Cholesterol: 0 mg; Carbohydrate: 22 gm;
Dietary Fiber: 0 gm; Protein: 2 gm; Sodium: 222 mg
Diabetic Exchanges: 1½ other carbohydrate

Preparation time: 10 minutes
Cooking time: 20 minutes
Total time: 30 minutes

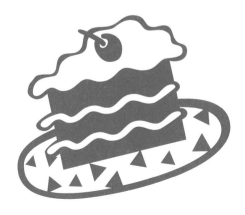

Strawberry Cream Trifle

Enjoy fresh strawberries that are gently nestled between layers of soft cake in a cloud of strawberry-flavored cream.

1 pound (½ quart) fresh strawberries, cleaned and sliced	1 cup ice cold water
½ cup Splenda Granular	1 (0.9-ounce) box sugar-free, fat-free banana cream pudding mix, dry
1 (0.32-ounce) box sugar-free strawberry-flavored gelatin, dry	1¾ cups skim milk
1 cup boiling water	1 (10.5-ounce) angel food cake, cut into thirds horizontally

- Gently toss the strawberries with the Splenda in a medium bowl and set aside.
- In another medium bowl stir the gelatin into 1 cup boiling water and stir for 2 minutes or until completely dissolved. Stir in 1 cup ice cold water (or 6 large ice cubes). Stir until the ice cubes are dissolved or until well mixed. Freeze for five minutes to soft-set the gelatin.
- In the meantime, in a third medium bowl mix the pudding and milk together with a mixer on medium speed for 2 minutes. Refrigerate for 5 minutes to soft-set.
- Arrange 1 layer of the angel food cake into the bottom of a trifle bowl. Tear 1 of the remaining layers of the angel food cake into pieces. Use half of the torn cake pieces to fill in any gaps between the layer of angel food cake that is currently in the trifle bowl and the trifle bowl itself. Also fill in the round hole in the middle of the cake. Set aside.
- Remove the gelatin and pudding from the freezer and refrigerator. Stir together until well blended. Gently stir in the sliced strawberries.
- Spoon half the strawberry mixture over the cake in the trifle bowl.

- Arrange the remaining angel food cake layer on top of the strawberry mixture and fill in the gaps with the remaining torn pieces of cake, just as you did for the first layer.
- Spoon the remaining strawberry mixture over the second layer of angel food cake.
- Cover and refrigerate for 2 to 3 hours or until completely set. Serve chilled.
- Garnish with additional fresh sliced strawberries if desired.

Yield: 20 ($^{1}/_{2}$-cup) servings

Calories: 61 (0% fat); Total Fat: 0 gm; Cholesterol: 0 mg; Carbohydrate: 13 gm;
Dietary Fiber: 1 gm; Protein: 2 gm; Sodium: 187 mg
Diabetic Exchanges: 1 other carbohydrate

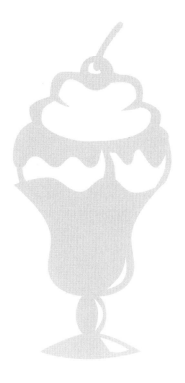 **Preparation time:** 20 minutes or less

Butterscotch Cream Dessert Dip

This creamy, smooth dessert topping tastes great on cakes, cupcakes, angel food cakes, or as filling in crêpes. It also makes a good dip with apples or peaches. Children enjoy dipping their fat-free animal crackers into them as well.

1 (1-ounce) package sugar-free butterscotch instant pudding mix, dry	1 (8-ounce) container fat-free dessert whipped topping
2 cups cold skim milk	2 tablespoons butterscotch chips, chopped into tiny pieces

- In a mixing bowl beat the pudding mix with the milk on medium speed for 2 minutes.
- Gently stir in the whipped topping and butterscotch pieces and keep stirring until well blended.
- Refrigerate until ready to serve.

Note: For Banana Cream Dessert Dip substitute sugar-free, fat-free banana cream instant pudding for the butterscotch pudding and omit the butterscotch chips.

Yield: 24 (2-tablespoon) servings

(with butterscotch pudding) Calories: 33 (11% fat); Total Fat: trace; Cholesterol: 0 mg; Carbohydrate: 6 gm; Dietary Fiber: 0 gm; Protein: 1 gm; Sodium: 66 mg Diabetic Exchanges: $1/2$ other carbohydrate
(with banana pudding) Calories: 26 (0% fat); Total Fat: 0 gm; Cholesterol: 0 mg; Carbohydrate: 5 gm; Dietary Fiber: 0 gm; Protein: 1 gm; Sodium: 65 mg Diabetic Exchanges: $1/2$ other carbohydrate

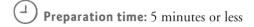 **Preparation time:** 5 minutes or less

Pumpkin & Ginger Snap Delight

Two thumbs up to Brenda Crosser who created this recipe! Brenda said in her notes to me that originally she created this recipe because she had leftover ginger snap cookies, but now she purposely purchases ginger snap cookies just so she can make this dessert!

16 ginger snap cookies, crushed*	4 cups fat-free, sugar-free frozen vanilla ice cream, softened
1 (1-ounce) box sugar-free, fat-free butterscotch pudding mix, dry	1 cup canned pumpkin
1/2 cup skim milk	1 teaspoon pumpkin pie spice

- Coat a 9 x 13-inch glass pan with nonfat cooking spray.
- Set aside 1/4 cup of the ginger snap cookie crumbs. Sprinkle the remaining crumbs on the bottom of the prepared pan.
- In a large mixing bowl mix the pudding mix and the milk together with an electric mixer until well blended and thick.
- Add the ice cream, pumpkin, and pumpkin pie spice and continue mixing until well blended. Pour over the cookie crumbs and spread evenly.
- Sprinkle the remaining ginger snap crumbs on top.
- Keep refrigerated until ready to eat. Do not freeze.
- If desired, top each serving with a dab of fat-free whipped topping.

Note: To make ginger snap crumbs, put the cookies into a plastic zip-top bag and seal shut while letting all the air out. Gently hit the sealed bag to crush the cookies with either the side of a 16-ounce can or a rolling pin.

Yield: 15 servings

Calories: 91 (12% fat); Total Fat: 1 gm; Cholesterol: 0 mg; Carbohydrate: 18 gm; Dietary Fiber: 1 gm; Protein: 2 gm; Sodium: 135 mg
Diabetic Exchanges: 1 other carbohydrate

Preparation time: 20 minutes or less

Pistachio Dream Dessert

I was so surprised at how super-refreshing and cool this dessert tasted. If you are in a pinch for a quickie dessert to serve right away, I suggest whipping this up and serving it in little dessert cups immediately after you make it, without even refrigerating. It is a fantastic and unique dessert!

2	(1-ounce) boxes sugar-free, fat-free pistachio pudding mix, dry	4	cups fat-free, sugar-free frozen vanilla ice cream, softened
1	cup skim milk		

- Coat a 9 x 13 glass casserole dish with nonfat cooking spray.
- In a large bowl mix the pudding mix and milk together with an electric mixer until well blended and thick.
- With an electric mixer, blend in the softened ice cream and continue mixing until well mixed.
- Spread the mixture into the prepared pan.
- Keep refrigerated until ready to eat. Do not freeze.

Yield: 15 servings

Calories: 63 (0% fat); Total Fat: 0 gm; Cholesterol: 0 mg; Carbohydrate: 14 gm; Dietary Fiber: 0 gm; Protein: 2 gm; Sodium: 191 mg
Diabetic Exchanges: 1 other carbohydrate

Preparation time: 15 minutes or less

Fudgesicle Dessert

This reminds me of a creamy "fudge cycle" on top of a thin cookie.

13$^{1}/_{2}$ squares chocolate graham crackers	4 cups no-sugar-added, reduced-fat vanilla ice cream
1$^{1}/_{2}$ cups cold water	2 tablespoons mini chocolate chips
2 (1.4-ounce) boxes sugar-free, fat-free instant chocolate pudding mix, dry	

- Arrange the graham crackers on the bottom of a 9 x 13-inch glass pan.
- In a large mixing bowl beat the water with the pudding mix with an electric mixer on medium speed until well blended and super thick.
- Continue beating and mix in the ice cream. Beat until well blended.
- Spread over the graham crackers.
- Sprinkle with the chocolate chips.
- Cover and keep refrigerated until ready to serve.

Yield: 16 servings

Calories: 92 (13% fat); Total Fat: 1 gm; Cholesterol: 0 mg; Carbohydrate: 18 gm; Dietary Fiber: 0 gm; Protein: 2 gm; Sodium: 252 mg
Diabetic Exchanges: 1 other carbohydrate

Preparation time: 10 minutes or less

Lemon Mousse Dessert

This super thick and creamy rich dessert will satisfy even the most finicky eaters who think they don't like diabetic desserts. One taste of this will change their minds!

1/2 cup graham cracker crumbs	2 quarts frozen low-fat vanilla yogurt, softened (I use Flavorite)
2 (I-ounce) boxes sugar-free, fat-free instant vanilla pudding mix, dry	2 teaspoons pure lemon extract
I cup cold water	

- Arrange the graham cracker crumbs on the bottom of a 9 x 13-inch glass pan.
- In a large mixing bowl beat the pudding mix with water with an electric mixer on medium speed until well blended and super thick.
- Continue beating and mix in the yogurt and lemon extract. Beat 2 or 3 minutes more or until well blended.
- Spread over the graham crackers.
- Serve immediately or cover and keep refrigerated until ready to serve.

Yield: 16 servings

Calories: 74 (21% fat); Total Fat: 2 gm; Cholesterol: 5 mg; Carbohydrate: 12 gm; Dietary Fiber: 0 gm; Protein: 3 gm; Sodium: 208 mg
Diabetic Exchanges: 1 other carbohydrate, 1/2 fat

Preparation time: 10 minutes or less

Mocha Mousse

This super rich and thick dessert is especially satisfying to coffee lovers.

4 **squares chocolate graham crackers, crushed**	1 **(2.1-ounce) box sugar-free, fat-free instant chocolate pudding mix, dry**
1 **cup brewed coffee, at room temperature or chilled**	1 **(8-ounce) container frozen fat-free whipped topping, thawed (I use Cool Whip)**

- Coat an 8-inch or 9-inch square pan with nonfat cooking spray. Set aside.
- Reserve 1 tablespoon graham cracker crumbs (to use as a decorative topping) and sprinkle the remaining graham cracker crumbs on the bottom of the pan. Set aside.
- In a medium mixing bowl beat together the coffee and pudding mix with an electric mixer until well blended and thick.
- Add the whipped topping and continue beating until well blended.
- Spread into the prepared pan.
- Sprinkle with the reserved graham cracker crumbs.
- Cover. Keep chilled until ready to serve.

Yield: 9 servings

Calories: 78 (7% fat); Total Fat: 1 gm; Cholesterol: 0 mg; Carbohydrate: 16 gm; Dietary Fiber: 0 gm; Protein: 0 gm; Sodium: 299 mg
Diabetic Exchanges: 1 other carbohydrate

Preparation time: 10 minutes or less

White Chocolate Mousse

This super thick mousse is a hit every time. My family loves it!

1 cup cold water	18 sprigs of mint for garnish (optional)
2 (1-ounce) boxes sugar-free, fat-free white chocolate instant pudding, dry	18 strawberries, sliced for garnish (optional)
1/2 gallon no-sugar-added, reduced-fat vanilla ice cream, softened	

- In a large mixing bowl beat the water with the pudding with an electric mixer until super thick.
- Continue beating and add the softened ice cream. Beat until well blended, thick, smooth, and creamy.
- Put 1/2 cup of the dessert into each dessert cup.
- Serve as is or keep refrigerated until ready to serve.
- Garnish with a sprig of fresh mint and a strawberry separated like a fan, if desired.

Yield: 18 (1/2-cup) servings

Calories: 85 (0% fat); Total Fat: 0 gm; Cholesterol: 0 mg; Carbohydrate: 19 gm;
Dietary Fiber: 0 gm; Protein: 3 gm; Sodium: 175 mg
Diabetic Exchanges: 1 1/2 other carbohydrate

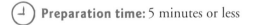 **Preparation time:** 5 minutes or less

Key Lime Dessert

This tangy dessert is an extra special treat if you thought you could no longer enjoy Key lime desserts in a diabetic lifestyle!

4	(0.3-ounce) boxes sugar-free lime gelatin, dry	2	(12-ounce) packages fat-free cream cheese, softened
4	cups boiling water	2	(10.5-ounce) angel food cakes, torn into 2-inch pieces
16	individual packets Splenda		

- Coat a springform pan or a 9 x 13-inch pan with nonfat cooking spray. Set aside.
- In a large bowl stir the gelatin into the boiling water until completely dissolved.
- With an electric mixer on low speed, mix the Splenda and cream cheese into the gelatin until completely dissolved and well mixed.
- Add the angel food cake pieces and continue mixing on low speed until all of the cake pieces are crumbled and are well mixed in with the gelatin.
- Pour into the prepared pan.
- Cover and refrigerate for 3 hours. Serve chilled.

Yield: 15 servings

Calories: 164 (0% fat); Total Fat: 0 gm; Cholesterol: 8 mg; Carbohydrate: 27 gm; Dietary Fiber: 1 gm; Protein: 10 gm; Sodium: 578 mg
Diabetic Exchanges: 2 other carbohydrate, 1 very lean meat

Preparation time: 10 minutes or less

Rainbow Trifle

This delightful dessert gets its name from the pretty layers of rainbow colors.

1	(0.3-ounce) box sugar-free lemon gelatin, dry	3	(8-ounce) packages fat-free cream cheese, softened
1	(0.32-ounce) box sugar-free raspberry gelatin, dry	2	(10.5-ounce) angel food cakes, cut into 1-inch pieces
1	(0.3-ounce) box sugar-free lime gelatin, dry	7	tablespoons finely chopped walnuts, divided

- Set out 3 large mixing bowls.
- Pour 1 cup of boiling water into each mixing bowl.
- Dissolve 1 envelope of gelatin into each bowl of boiling water and stir until completely dissolved.
- Dissolve 1 package of cream cheese into each of the bowls of gelatin. With a mixer on medium speed, mix the cream cheese into the gelatin water until smooth.
- Divide the cake pieces evenly among the 3 bowls of gelatin. Add 2 tablespoons of the nuts to each bowl. Gently stir until the gelatin mixture is absorbed.
- Refrigerate all 3 bowls for about 10 minutes or until slightly set.
- Gently spoon the lime cake mixture into the bottom of a trifle bowl or large glass bowl. Do not press. You want to be able to see the chunks of cake.
- Gently spoon the raspberry cake mixture over the lime. Do not press.
- Gently spoon the lemon cake mixture over the raspberry. Do not press.
- Sprinkle the remaining 1 tablespoon nuts over the lemon cake mixture.
- Cover and refrigerate for at least 1 hour or until completely chilled. I think the longer it is chilled the better it tastes.

Yield: 24 ($\frac{1}{2}$-cup) servings

Calories: 224 (14% fat); Total Fat: 3 gm; Cholesterol: 10 mg; Carbohydrate: 33 gm;
Dietary Fiber: 1 gm; Protein: 13 gm; Sodium: 707 mg
Diabetic Exchanges: 2 other carbohydrate, 2 very lean meat

Fruit Dip

Brenda Crosser sent in this versatile dip. She used it for fruit.

I	(I-ounce) box sugar-free, fat-free vanilla instant pudding mix, dry	I	tablespoon Splenda Granular
		I	teaspoon vanilla extract
2¹/₂	cups fat-free half-and-half	I	teaspoon almond extract

- In a mixing bowl, with an electric mixer beat the pudding mix, half-and-half, Splenda, vanilla extract, and almond extract on medium speed for 2 minutes.
- Ready to eat as is or keep chilled until ready to eat.

Yield: 20 (2-tablespoon) servings

Calories: 26 (0% fat); Total Fat: 0 gm; Cholesterol: 0 mg; Carbohydrate: 5 gm; Dietary Fiber: 0 gm; Protein: 2 gm; Sodium: 89 mg
Diabetic Exchanges: ¹/₂ other carbohydrate

Preparation time: 5 minutes or less

INDEX

About the Author

Entrepreneur of Cozy Homestead Publishing, Dawn Hall self-published her first cookbook in 1996 to raise money for her husband's brain cancer treatments and since then has sold over 750,000 copies (even though she didn't know how to type, use a computer, or anything about publishing). Today, she is the award-winning author of the Busy People's cookbooks: *Busy People's Slow Cooker Cookbook, Busy People's Low-Fat Cookbook,* and *Busy People's Down-Home Cooking Without the Down-Home Fat.*

Dawn is a successful recovering compulsive overeater and food addict. She was born watching her weight. With over ten years of experience as an accomplished aerobic instructor and facilitator for W.O.W. (Watching Our Weight), Dawn walks her talk and is living proof that you can have your cake and eat it too.

She strongly believes her talent for creating extremely low-fat, mouth-watering foods that are made quickly and effortlessly is a gift from God. As a way of saying thank you a portion of her profits from this book go to Christian Health Ministries.

Dawn is a popular inspirational speaker and veteran talk show guest. She has appeared on the *700 Club*, CBN, *Woman to Woman, Good Morning A.M., Life Today with James Robison,* along with numerous other T.V. and radio programs nationwide. You can visit her website at www.DawnHallCookbooks.com. To contact her, call, write, or fax:

Cozy Homestead Publishing
c/o Dawn Hall
5425 S. Fulton-Lucas Road
Swanton, OH 43558
(419) 826-2665 or fax (419) 825-2700
Dawn@DawnHallCookbooks.com

Christian Health Ministries

A portion of the proceeds from this cookbook go to help Christian Health Ministries in Toledo, Ohio. It is a nonprofit organization of volunteer doctors and nurses who offer basic health care to the working poor free of charge.

They are in constant need of volunteers. For more information contact:

Christian Health Ministries,
1630 Broadway
Toledo, Ohio 43609
(419) 243-5371
ChristianDocs@aol.com
Requests4Healing@aol.com

———

I believe strongly that my cookbooks are a gift from God and were used to help pay for my loving first husband's medical treatments for brain cancer I want to continue using my cookbooks to help others in need with their medical expenses.

My publisher graciously permits me to allow others with uncovered medical expenses to use all of my cookbooks as fundraisers. If you are interested in holding a fundraiser using any of my cookbooks please, go to my website at: http://www.dawnhallcookbooks.com for more information.

Book for a Buck

If you would like a receive a free copy of *The Message of Hope* with information on how to have a personal relationship with God so that you can have more love, joy, and peace in your life send $1.00 to help cover postage to: Cozy Homestead, 5425 South Fulton-Lucas Road., Swanton, Ohio, 43558.